PLAGUE OR PSEUDO PLAGUE 2021

Hugh Cameron MB ChB FRCS(C)

Library of Congress Control Number:		2022902612
ISBN:	Hardcover	978-1-6698-1064-3
	Softcover	978-1-6698-1063-6
	eBook	978-1-6698-1062-9

Print information available on the last page.

Rev. date: 02/08/2022

To order additional copies of this book, contact:
Xlibris
844-714-8691
www.Xlibris.com
Orders@Xlibris.com
837897

Contents

Introduction ... ix
Lessons From The Past ... xiii

January 1 ... 1
January 6 ... 3
January 15 ... 6
January 26 at 4:33 PM ... 8
January 30 at 2:00 PM ... 11
February 2 at 2:01 PM ... 13
February 6 at 8:08 PM ... 15
February 10 at 1:47 PM ... 17
February 12 at 5:06 PM ... 19
February 15 at 3:57 PM ... 21
February 18 at 9:28 PM ... 23
February 23 at 12:20 PM ... 25
February 25 at 3:42 PM ... 28
March 1 at 6:30 PM ... 30
March 6 at 3:00 PM ... 32
March 9 at 4:44 PM ... 35
March 14 at 6:27 PM ... 37
March 18 at 5:54 PM ... 40
March 22 at 5:09 PM ... 42
March 25 at 3:50 PM ... 44
March 30 at 6:24 PM ... 46
April 4 at 7:00 PM ... 49
April 8 at 4:58 PM ... 52
April 12 at 5:14 PM ... 55
April 17 at 2:26 PM ... 58
April 21 at 5:05 PM ... 61
April 24 at 12:38 PM ... 63

April 28 at 12:19 PM 65
May 1 67
May 5 69
May 10 71
May 14....................73
May 20 75
May 24 77
May 29 79
June 3....................81
June 7....................84
June 12....................86
June 16....................89
June 21....................91
June 27....................93
July 4....................95
July 10....................97
July 16 at 8:15 PM....................100
July 22 at 10:50 PM....................103
July 29 at 4:04 PM 106
August 4 at 3:35 PM 109
August 11 at 5:27 PM 112
August 16 at 5:12 PM 114
August 20 at 5:25 PM....................116
August 24 at 3:18 PM 118
August 28 at 11:24 AM 121
September 3 at 5:15 PM....................123
September 8 at 10:40 PM....................125
September 10 at 5:39 PM....................127
September 15 at 4:07 PM....................130
September 19 at 6:33 PM....................132
September 24 at 6:24 PM....................135
October 1 at 7:56 PM....................138
October 6 at 6:35 PM....................141
October 11 at 6:01 PM....................144
October 16 at 11:34 AM 147
October 20 at 5:20 PM 150
October 23 at 12:34 PM 152
October 26 at 4:27 PM 155

October 30 at 1:17 PM 158
November 5 at 4:51 PM 161
November 10 at 1:33 PM 163
November 14 at 6:08 PM 165
November 16 at 1:49 PM 167
November 18 at 5:21 PM 168
November 20 at 11:37 AM 170
November 22 at 4:06 PM 172
November 26 at 4:45 PM 174
November 30 at 3:59 PM 176
December 5 at 6:43 PM 178
December 11 at 12:07 PM 180
December 15 at 3:53 PM 182
December 21 at 6:21 PM 184
December 23 at 5:35 PM 186
December 27 at 10 PM 188
December 29 At 5 PM 190

Envoi 191
Acknowledgements 193

Introduction

'Heaven and earth have no pity; they regard all things as straw dogs'. Lao-tsz 550 BC. Perhaps the last year has shown that pity and compassion can be a scarce phenomenon.

My first book on the Wuhan virus, in what sadly seems destined to become a series, was entitled the Journal of the Plague Year (2020). It was originally a collection of sequential posts which began when the virus erupted in the West. Many of these posts were penned as requests of friends and patients for information about the virus, as what was available in the legacy media and pundits with unsavory connections, was contradictory, frequently clearly inaccurate, and occasionally ludicrously wrong.

While I am an orthopedic surgeon and not a virologist, I have an extensive background in science. As an airborne respiratory virus epidemic is hardly quantum physics, some of the pronouncements from 'so-called' experts clearly made no sense at all and showed a frightening lack of knowledge. Many of these 'experts' were incredibly narrowly focused on a single incident and absolutely failed to look at the overall picture, with predictably disastrous results.

The situation darkened when innocuous posts started to be deleted by so-called 'fact checkers,' who turned out to be people with dubious sources of funding, political ideologies, and with clearly often little knowledge at all about medicine or science.

Some research papers, rushed into publication, in what used to be very reputable journals, were so clearly untrue that they could not be explained on the basis of careless science. No one who publishes in a reputable journal is that bad, and no journal who wishes to retain any credibility would publish such obvious untruths. And yet it was happening, not only in one journal, but across the board. Some journals later recanted, but why allow such clear anti-science propaganda in the first case?

Some of my posts were disappearing and occasionally reappearing when challenged, so I became alarmed that history was being rewritten, Soviet style, before our very eyes. I felt that the only way to ensure that there was some sort of archival record of what had actually happened was to publish in book form. Which I did in January of 2021.

Initially I thought that the clear mishandling of this epidemic was due to the desperation exhibited by the media and others trying to unseat the US president. Once they had achieved their objective I thought that the US, if nowhere else, would return to sanity. Sadly, that did not happen, so the root cause of this tsunami of false data and inexplicable mandates was obviously deeper, although US politics clearly played a role.

The situation got even darker as more and more censorship appeared, with the frightening spectacle of extremely reputable scientists being silenced in social media. Mandates grew more and more fantastical, with clearly no basis in reality. Given this breakdown of legitimate information and thought, It became obvious that a second book recording this inexplicable ongoing man-made tragedy would be required.

As before, this book consists of virtually unedited sequential posts to give continuity to the history of this strange time as it emerged. Also included are some very penetrating observations by readers, for whose comments I am grateful.

Due to the fear of fact checking censors and algorithms, proper names have very seldom been used. I found almost eighteen months ago that the mention of Ai Fen, the Chinese doctor who tried to warn the world, resulted in the instant removal of the post. In Canada unbelievably, our doctor's licensing bodies insisted, in writing, that official guidelines regarding lock down, etc. and in particular vaccines, must be followed without question, under threat of loss of medical license if we deviate from the party line.

It has therefore been necessary to call the vaccine, the needle, or a similar term, and even then be extremely circumspect. Drugs used to great effect in other countries similarly cannot be spoken of in Canada or on social media. The names of well-known doctors brought immediate censorship so I have used their first names only in almost all cases.

The worldwide protests finally underway in most countries rejecting lockdown and various vaccine mandates may indicate that freedom is at least in sight. The fact that the legacy media and politicians are completely ignoring such events does not bode well, however. It must be remembered that 200 Bolsheviks took over Russia in 1917 and held Eastern Europe in prison for 70 years, and Cuba, China, North Korea, and Venezuela remain under collectivist totalitarian rule.

In editing this book the publisher has insisted I remove the names of all people and all drugs. This is in spite of the fact that these are posts published in FB. I have had to comply.

Lessons From The Past

I am an orthopedic surgeon, and an expert in various narrow fields such as bioengineering, joint replacement and pain. The classic definition of an expert is one who knows more and more about less and less. Until I stopped operating a couple of years ago and returned to general orthopedics, my focus was so narrow I knew little and cared less about what was going on in the rest of medicine outside orthopedics and had a passing interest only in the rest of the world.

The Legacy Media I had abandoned decades ago, when I found that everything which they reported which I actually knew about, bore no relation to the facts. TV was even worse. Mine broke about ten years ago and I never had it repaired. So I was blissfully unaware of what was happening, outside my own small field. And this was in spite of the fact I was traveling all over the world, teaching, and demonstrating joint replacement. At one time I had in excess of a million complementary air miles. I learned how to go to Australia for the day. All this I described in a light hearted autobiography entitled Have Knife Will Travel.

What this meant was that I had a certain naivety. For example, I believed in Big Pharma. Having worked in a university for most of my life, I had seen the collapse of these institutions as the administrative class gradually took over. Research grants, which used to go to the researcher, had progressively to be shared with the administrators, as there were more and more of them. Why they were there and what they did with their time, other than make up utterly pointless rules, was never clear to me.

It all happened so slowly that I never found a hill to die on. Eventually, with Edna Quammie, my long term scrub nurse and friend, I documented our observations on this slow moving tragedy in our book, 'The Big House. Toronto General Hospital from 1972 to 1984.'

I knew that major advances in medications no longer came from universities. Almost all that is done there is 'me too' research, as it is so difficult to get any radically new concept or idea through the university or hospital review boards. These committees are staffed with has-beens and never-wasses, professional bench-warmers. But without their permission, nothing can be done. In universities little that is fundamentally new has been done in the last decade or two. So I defended Big Pharma as the producer of all new medications.

For years all I knew came from conversations with friends all over the world, and occasionally newspapers lying around airport lounges. That was enough for me. I resisted getting a cell phone. I got one when they first came out, but people kept phoning me so I got rid of it. If they wanted to speak to me they could speak to my secretary and she could decide. Eventually, a couple of years ago a US friend, for whom I consult, demanded I get a cell phone, so my son gave me his old one.

It was magic. It opened up a whole new world I had no idea existed. I was entranced. I could listen on my phone to some of the greatest thinkers in the world. Not only present, but past. I was totally uninterested in politics or in the most recent scares, as news after all is 'man bites dog', not 'dog bites man'.

I had known virtually since the inception that man-made global warming was a scam as I knew the idea had been floated by the prime minister of Sweden decades ago, along with the scares like holes in the ozone layer, lake acidification, etc. I also knew of the player who, after wrecking energy production in Ontario, Canada, really got the ball rolling at the UN, probably or possibly ultimately with the backing of China.

I knew nothing about these computer modelers, who pretended to model diseases. I knew of course, as everyone with even a passing interest knew, that the so-called global warming climate modelers, except possibly the Russians, were producing fantasies, doubtless for their own ends.

Climategate showed that what they were producing was not factual, and that they knew it was not factual. The tragedy was that the world ignored that and carried on merrily with the myth of man-made global warming. In a sense, that was the end of science which could be trusted. From then on no scientific statement could be taken at face value.

So this was the scene when the Wuhan virus was released. We now know it probably escaped from a lab in Wuhan, in May of 2019. It was probably spread deliberately at the International Military Games in Wuhan in October of 2019, and further reinforced during the diaspora in the Chinese Lunar New Year, when flights inside China were banned but international flights encouraged, with the assistance of the corrupt WHO.

Nothing much happened initially. The virus quietly spread as respiratory viruses always do and then responded to a seasonal trigger, which we don't yet understand, and the number of cases rocketed up. By March of 2020, we were hearing figures of 3% mortality and that the Bat Woman of Wuhan had added HIV taken from the level 4 lab in Winnipeg, Canada. If so, there would be no immunity ever and a large percentage of the world's population would die.

It was at this point I began to write what ended up as a Journal of the Plague Year 2020, as I kept getting questions from my patients and friends all over the world. That book documented a doctor's journey from fear to relief when we found that if HIV had been added it was inactive, to utter disbelief when universal masking was introduced in the middle of the summer of 2020, when there were virtually no deaths, and the fear was kept going solely on the basis of the misused PCR test. The developer of the concept behind the test, who got the Nobel prize for it, said it was never to be used in that way. His advice was ignored.

The main institutions on which the whole world had trusted fell one by one. WHO was obviously simply a willing tool of the CCP. The CDC in the US soon also gave every evidence of corruption or incompetence as did the FDA. But even WHO, looking at the devastation being produced in the Third World by CCP inspired lockdown, felt they could not continue to countenance this charade, reversed themselves and declared that it should cease.

Unfortunately by this time the rest of the world had bought into and seemed to like lockdown. The politicians loved it, some for very obvious political non-medical reasons. So it continued, fueled mainly by so-called cases of positive PCR tests. Eventually even the CDC admitted that that test was all but useless. As it was such a handy instrument to control the populace by inducing fear, it's use continued and the Legacy media and Public Health personnel kept reporting positive tests as if they meant something.

So with that introduction to the ongoing worldwide charade, of a lethal virus which was effectively a risk to the ill elderly only, a new year begins. Anno Domine 2021.

January 1

Happy New Year! Really? To quote Julius Caesar, 'a year older, and no wiser, and the crowds along the Appian Way remain the same.' That reality seems to me best expressed by David Hume (1750), the only philosopher I really liked; 'nothing is more surprising than the ease with which the many are governed by the few.'

We are still no nearer to understanding the Wuhan virus. We more or less accept that it came from the Wuhan lab and the target was the nonproductive ill elderly. Whether it's escape was deliberate or an error, remains unknown. As no government or organization seems prepared to hold anyone to account, it really doesn't matter.

After it escaped, it was spread deliberately through the world. As there appears to be no penalty for doing so, one wonders when the next one will appear. This was evil, but perfectly understandable. It is the reaction of the rest of the world which was not.

All the experience, and all Western science in the handling of epidemics, which was outlined by WHO in the fall of 2019, was suddenly tossed aside in 2020 by WHO and the CDC. Obviously one had been suborned, but the other? And, with the exception of Sweden, Brazil, and Belarus, why did the rest of the world follow?

Maybe it was simply panic. But the outbreak on the Diamond Princess cruise ship was a perfect laboratory experiment, so we knew the virus was not so deadly. We knew by spring of 2020 that it was the ill elderly who were the targets. So lockdown was counterproductive, making this group more vulnerable, not less. And yet lockdown persists. And mandatory masking in the middle of summer for a seasonal virus, when there were virtually no deaths, was inexplicable. We knew it made no sense then and a recent study from Denmark has confirmed that.

Even stranger was the banning of drugs which had been shown to be of some value. These were drugs with a long track record and were available over the counter in many countries. Even if they weren't that effective, why criminalize them? I, as an interested doc, only heard about one of these drugs in the summer of 2020. How very odd. Even mention of these drugs will get a post censored.

One doesn't want to overstate the case, but it is starting to sound like the Soviet Union described by Alexander Solzhenitsyn, the Russian, and Milan Kundera, the Czech writer, where it is off to the gulag for telling a joke. Victor Hugo (1870), wrote that 'invasion of armies is resisted; the invasion of ideas is not.' One feels that there is something terribly wrong. Maybe the safest thing to do is shut up and follow the example of the Pharisee and 'pass by on the other side.'

But when one wonders what sort of world we will be leaving our children, one has to feel like Goethe (1820). 'Du kannst, denn du sollst.' 'You can, for you must.' So we have to keep trying to see our way out of this disaster.

Q,1. I hear that Vitamin D is useful.

A,1. I hear the same thing. I used to take 1,000 iu per day. But now I hear that in northern countries like Canada we need 4,000 iu per day in the winter, which lasts most of the year. Half an hour in the summer sun gives a similar dose.

Q,2. Should we be afraid to take the vaccine? I'm really confused and conflicted about this.

A,2. If you are under 60 and probably under 70, if you are healthy, I don't see any reason to take the vaccine. Certainly no healthy child needs it.

January 6

'Strange friend,' said I. 'Here is no cause to mourn.'
'None,' said the other, 'Save the undone years,
the hopelessness.' Wilfred Owen 1918.

The world mismanagement of the Wuhan virus remains a mystery. Several years ago, WHO changed the definition of a Pandemic to 'a disease present in a whole country or world.' The word 'lethal' was removed. This means that any time, any politician can declare seasonal flu a Pandemic and order a lockdown.

The WHO guidelines in 2019 cautioned against quarantine and mandatory masking. The concept of lockdown was so ludicrous it was not mentioned. In 2020, suddenly everything changed and WHO and the CDC and then the rest of the world began to follow Chinese Communist ideas. WHO has since reverted to the 2019 guidelines, at least regarding the futility and harmful effects of lockdown, but not the rest of the world.

One of the problems is lack of reliable data. The PCR test was used in a manner the developer said it should not be. When run at a 37x multiplier it is practically guaranteed to pick up a piece of a dead virus. So a PCR positive test, which is all the legacy media reports, is meaningless. The only thing worth looking at is the death rate, recognizing that this is also grossly exaggerated. The CDC in America changed the death reporting so that anyone who died with the virus was reported as dying of the virus. They have since admitted to this willful exaggeration.

It is possible to get data from the net. If you look at the excess deaths by year, 2020 is not much different than previous years. If the excess winter respiratory deaths are down one year they will be up the next, as more susceptible people are around.

Similarly if you look at a Gompertz curve of virus deaths in all countries, you really can't tell them apart, other than northern and southern hemispheres. The curves showed no change with lockdown, masking, and the rest. The curve for Sweden with no lockdown is the same and seems to be doing better in the expected winter resurgence than countries with severe lockdown.

Looking at the momentous events of history like WW1, there is a similar pattern. The useless generals ordered young men, the flower of Europe, to charge into machine guns. This was done in the US civil war against the Gatling gun and in the last battle in the Satsuma samurai rebellion in 1877. If interested, see the movie, The Last Samurai. So the WW1 generals must have known and yet they ordered it, and Europe died. Art died, poetry died, music died, architecture died, religion died. Hard to believe that even the stupid could be so stupid. But it was surely not planned!

But yet, there is this ongoing lockdown which is destroying the economies of the West. The small businesses are going under never to return.

I was thinking of publishing my posts of last year, after the fashion of Daniel Defoe's book, Journal of a Plague Year (1722), detailing the change from the sense of doom, to hope, to relief that it was over, and then puzzlement when mandatory masking came in when a seasonal virus had passed through and there were no deaths, to disbelief, and then a feeling of despair. I would like to thank those who shared their thoughts of this strange journey. It makes W.B.Yeats sound prophetic,

'Things fall apart; the center cannot hold.
The best lack all conviction, while the worst
are full of passionate intensity.
The darkness drops again,
and the rough beast, it's hour come at last,
slouches to Davos to be born.'

Q.1. A year ago the Canadian government paid off the mainstream media with $600 million of our tax dollars. I am very concerned that people are unaware of this and are thus believing their distorted stories. There is no real journalism any more.

Q,2. WHO and CDC have recently changed the definition of herd immunity to read 'when a sufficient number of people have been vaccinated.' They are trying to make vaccination mandatory.

Q,3. I listened to the German bacteriologist. Very interesting and very worrying.

Q,4. Bureaucrats, Autocrats, Aristocrats; beware of the crats!

A. All these comments are very true. Dr S is well worth listening to, with considerable concern. He described the problem with blood clots, especially in the brain, induced by the vaccine. It subsequently turned out that he was right. The full history of this has yet to be written. Certainly truth and the legacy media have only a fleeting contact.

January 15

'Come let us sit upon the ground and tell sad stories of the death of kings.' Shakespeare (Richard 11). The winds of change have turned into a hurricane. The voices of dissent are vanishing, leaving an eerie silence.

It is no longer safe to take any position not held by those who control the legacy media. The guillotine is raised or 'the swords await at the tent door'. Maybe it is time to pack our bags and gently steal away; to find some safe haven and hunker down until the storm has passed. But where and for how long?

The Winter Palace in St. Petersburg was stormed in 1917 ushering in the reign of terror which lasted 70 years, until the fall of the Berlin Wall in 1989.

I was lecturing in Braunschweig, a few klicks from that border, the night the people of East Germany finally had enough and brought down that symbol of monstrous tyranny. About 2 million East Germans came across the border that night. I remember the silence and the profound sense of relief that the long nightmare was over. Francis Fukuyama published a book entitled The End Of History in 2014, believing that freedom and democracy would liberate the whole world. Sadly, we were all mistaken.

The lights went out in Rome in AD 455 and the Dark Ages descended. There were some rumblings of freedom with the signing of the Magna Carta in 1215. But it was not until 1700 that the Enlightenment exploded upon the world; that strange concept that each individual was an individual, not part of a hive or a collective.

The Enlightenment has lasted 300 years, a mere blink of an eye in the great sweep of history. In the last decade it has been fading like morning dew. Then came the virus, a tightly targeted virus which produced an extraordinary response, and it all came crashing down. Kipling wrote,

'Gone, gone, gone with Thebes the Golden,
don't tell me now I didn't give you warning.'

Will the hopes and dreams of the Enlightenment return? Who knows! Stranger things have happened. The West won, against all odds, at Marathon, Actium, Tours, Vienna, and Lepanto. So maybe, as Francis Thompson wrote,

'is my gloom after all, shade of his hand
outstretched caressingly?'

Q,1. I keep hoping perhaps the populace will one day awaken and see reality. If they don't, I am rather glad to be the age I am as I won't see the destruction of all the hopes of the world. My offspring and theirs will, and that saddens me.

A,1. Deus Vult, God willing, sanity and the ideas of the Enlightenment will return. But currently they are missing in action.

January 26 at 4:33 PM

'From the fury of the Vikings may the good Lord protect us,' was the prayer of the English monks. Nowadays, for the hapless users of Social Media, the prayer is to 'protect us from the fury of the algorithm.' With so many experts disappearing or being made to disappear, one is frightened to put pen to paper in case one comes to the notice of those avatars of truth, the fact checkers.

It is no longer clear which facts one dare mention. I thought lockdown would end in the US in November, but I am pleased to see that it is finally being lifted, at least partially, even in some of the most doctrinaire states, in spite of the rising numbers of actual cases. This is of course winter when respiratory and seasonal virus infections and deaths spike.

It remains difficult to get reliable data. Most people now know that the CDC changed the definition last spring so that deaths possibly with the virus, no matter how remote, were called deaths of the virus. Their numbers therefore are grossly exaggerated and completely irrelevant. It was just as bad in the UK, and in many other countries with a death within 30 days of a positive test being called a virus death. Almost everyone now knows that the PCR test, run at a 37x multiplier, is largely meaningless. I do hear whispers that it is going to be reduced to 20x when a positive test may mean an actual infection.

The only truly accurate figures are excess deaths, that is the number who died over the expected deaths, compared year to year. In some countries we know that there have been little or no excess deaths, so where is the epidemic?

Data from the trials of the magic jab are difficult to find, including the criteria for success or even diagnosis. In my hospital we all have to take the flu vaccine every year, or wear a mask all winter, all the time. But strangely, not this year. So far they have not insisted, but I am sure once they have adequate supplies of the vaccine they will. I am of an age where the immune response is low, so I don't think I am at risk of a vaccine induced cytokine storm.

My sister in law, is busy giving AZ jabs by the hundreds in England. She says that other than a sore arm and flu-like symptoms her patients have been OK. They don't vaccinate anyone with a history of allergies or a positive PCR test within a month. (If someone has actually had the disease they don't need a vaccination. So obviously the fact that these PCR positive people are being vaccinated at all means the authorities in England don't actually believe that a positive PCR test means anything.)

As I feared, lockdown in many countries and universal masking will continue until spring when the virus will go away as it did last year. They will then claim that lockdown and masking saved the world.

And so we wait for spring when people can come out of their bunkers and look at a ruined world. As T.S. Elliot wrote, 'in the juvescence of the year came Christ the tiger.' The small business person will see everything they had worked for, all gone. 'Gone, gone, gone with lost Atlantis.' I foresee a tidal wave of deaths of despair.

Q,1. Read C.S. Lewis "Old Devil's Letter to the Young.' 1942. Sound familiar?

A,1. I did read that book, and she is right! Plus ça change, plus c'est la même chose! C.S. Lewis describes our current situation exactly. I can't reproduce it here because of copyright, but I certainly recommend reading it. It will make your blood run cold. It is such an accurate description.

Q,2. I was worried you had been silenced. The fury of the algorithm made me chuckle because it is true. I often misspell words and names purposefully to fool it.

A,2. I became aware of how much censoring was going on last year. I mentioned Ai Fen, the heroic doctor in Wuhan who first tried to alert the world about this virus. That post was taken down. Since then I have avoided using names in case they are retroactively disappeared as people were in the Soviet Union.

Patients in Canada and the US are being told that there is no treatment, so go home and hide there. When you turn blue and are dying, come to a hospital. This is the first time I am aware of in the West when treatment, which has proved successful, is forbidden by a government. Why it should be forbidden remains unknown.

January 30 at 2:00 PM

'Is there no help for the widow's son?' Now the election in the US is finally over, lockdown is being lifted. I hear that the PCR test is going to be reduced from a 37x multiplier, which practically guarantees to find a bit of dead virus from the next street over, to 20x, which if positive, means that you probably have the virus, even if like many people, you have no symptoms.

I thought that the virus would vanish in the US in November but the political uncertainty kept the fear machine in action until now. The survivors can now come out and look around at a ruined world. My father, a padre in the 51st Highland Division (or I think that is what it was, as men of his generation seldom talked about their experiences in the war), told me about coming through the bombed out, ruined German cities as the war was ending; the sense of desolation. But at least they had the US Marshall plan to rebuild. Today, there is no Marshall plan. With the proposed destruction of cheap energy and manufacturing, due to the push for the 'Green New Deal', the Western world seems to be going the opposite way.

This strange universal masking persists with the sainted Dr suggesting double masking. There never was any evidence for it in the first place and I thought that the Danish study had eventually dispelled that fairy tale. Oh well, in the US it is only for another 100 days or until Joe forgets his edict.

In Canada and the rest of the world the inexplicable behavior persists. We have new travel restrictions, in spite of the fact that the documented transmission from travel is 1.8%, only a little above bars and restaurants at 1.4%. To keep out this new version I suppose. But a virus mutates to become more infectious and less deadly. Yes!! Less deadly, otherwise it dies out by killing the host.

One PHJ in Canada wants to stop the March break because there will be more cases. Spring is coming and this is a seasonal virus so I doubt that. But I am in favor of stopping school holidays. The original reason for summer holidays was that the kids could help on the farm. There are no farms in Toronto, and the kids have got to catch up for the lost year.

Finally some of the younger people have had enough, with anti-lockdown riots in Spain, Holland, and Denmark. A few hundred years ago the Danes were the fierce ones, with the Viking ships landing and the spear Danes and sword Danes rushing up the beach. But then that went away. The thought of the docile Danes rioting means that there is hope for the world.

Hopefully the young people will no longer accept what has been done to them. They have been crucified for the last year on a cross of media driven fear for a condition which never affected them. Maybe they have begun to stand up. Maybe there is hope for the widow's son.

Q,1. This is being pushed for money, mainly mass vaccinations. Just look at the business model. It went from a multimillion dollar a year industry to a multi trillion dollar industry. Get everyone to take 2 or 3 shots a year forever. No liability if they get injured. And then you sell them the drugs to treat the injury. What a great business model!

Q,2. Why is only the PCR test available in most places?

A,1. From a reader, which I think is accurate, this inexplicable policy is being driven by 'power, money and control'. I can't think of any other reason.

Q,3. The death rate for the healthy under 60 or really under 70 is so low, why vaccinate, especially children?

A,2. From another reader, the same answer, 'too much power, money and control.' Hard to think of any other explanation.

February 2 at 2:01 PM

The young, who have been in chains for almost a year now for a condition which never affected them, must feel like Johnnie Armstrong, the captured Scottish rustler, when he was appealing King James for clemency.

'To seek hot water beneath cold ice,
surely it is a great folly.
I have sought grace from a graceless face,
but there is none for my men and me.'

It looks as if governments around the world have no intention of freeing the young until every living thing has had the vac. My sister in law in England, giving out jabs by the hundreds, says that even those who tested positive are being jabbed. We now know that those who have had the virus are immune. The fear initially was that Bat Woman had added HIV. In May 2020, the Koreans, who I trust, confirmed that if she had added HIV, it was inactive, so if you get the disease you are immune. So if the authorities in the UK are mandating jabs after a positive PCR, it means that they don't believe that the PCR test means anything. In other words, fuhgeddaboudit, other than someone is making real money from these worthless tests.

Laura from England, a clever woman I heard this morning, points out that even if you fall off a cliff, the dead body may contain a trace of virus, so, given the current reporting, you will have died of the virus. This means that they can claim people are dying and so continue to mandate a jab every week or month or year, forever, as the virus mutates a little.

The Alice in Wonderland logic continues. In Ontario skiing causes the virus. How this could be only a government man would understand.

Similarly, you cannot fly from Canada to Mexico or the Caribbean. What this ban is supposed to do is not clear. If you want to go, fly to the US and then fly from there to Mexico.

Schools are still closed in Canada. They are open in most of the rest of the world, but teachers unions continue to fight to keep them closed. The teachers clearly see schools as being there for their benefit and the children are simply a nuisance. Universities are similar. Take the money and forget the teaching. Given that virtually no history or literature is taught anyway, that might not be so bad. No ideas are better than bad ideas.

Shakespeare and Chaucer are no longer taught, and in some places, the greatest American novel, Gone With The Wind, has been banned. That achingly beautiful book was the inspiration for my own serial novel, To Slip the Surly Bonds of Earth. The fourth in that series, Redemption, has just been published, and the first two are available in audiobook. If they can ban Gone With The Wind, what can't they ban?

Sadly it looks as if the freedom of the West has also gone with the wind.

Q,1. The totalitarians are brilliant strategists...it is only their useful idiots who are brainless.

Q,2. The media have done a stellar job terrifying people.

Q,3. You must have faith. Why do you think they have closed the churches? That is what the communists did.

Q,4. Nothing government is working in Toronto. So why do we still have to pay taxes?

Q,5. The subway is not working in Toronto and the buses are jammed. Where is the social distancing? If we can't socially distance on a government bus, why are restaurants closed?

Q, 6. I looked at my child's zoom class. Not much teaching going on there.

A,1. What can you say? Every single one of these points from readers is valid. Clearly no one who thinks for themselves is buying this government disinformation.

February 6 at 8:08 PM

'Plus ça change, plus c'est la même chose', or 'things change but remain the same.' Or so it seems from reviewing the legacy media and the edicts of the Public Health Johnnies (PHJs). Talleyrand (1820) described both as having 'learned nothing and forgotten nothing.' The Chinese communist inspired lockdown and mandatory masking remain their only idea. They fail to understand what Virgil (30 BC) wrote, 'sunt lacrimae rerum,' or 'events have tears'.

The PHJs and the media still breathlessly report positive PCR cases as if this meant something. Everyone now knows just how that one works. Even mortality rates are meaningless, as if a death occurs within a month or more of finding a trace of dead virus, the death is labeled as COVID. Similarly, the actual diagnosis of why someone was in the ICU in the first place doesn't matter if there is a trace of virus after they have been admitted..

Quod est veritas? What is truth? asked Pontius Pilate. Years from now, our kids, who have been fed this terrifying story that they will die of the virus or the earth going up in flames, are going to ask why were they told these lies? They will assume everything is a lie and believe nothing.

'Truth is a dagger in the hand of a child.' I can't remember where that quotation came from, but those running social media certainly seem to believe it. Reality, the virus, and global warming are very far apart.

Will sanity ever return, or is this simply the last gasp of Western civilization? Universities and public education have been trying now for a couple of generations to undermine the Enlightenment, that strange and unlikely concept that individuals are individuals and have some intrinsic value. They have sought a return to the hive, the collective, where there are no individuals, simply groups.

This is 2021 so it is hard to believe that the Holodomor of the Ukraine or The Great Hunger of China is coming. But it did not take long to change Venezuela from the richest country in South America to a country where it is illegal to put 'starvation' as a cause of death on a child's death certificate.

Surely not, surely this is just a bad dream, and everything will be just fine. Tomorrow is another day!

Q,1. You sound rather negative tonight. I think we must maintain the hope that sanity will eventually prevail somewhere, in many minds. There is a feeling of unrest. More and more people are speaking out. Hope is alive.

A,1. I am sure you are right. Hold the faith. As Henley wrote

'Out of the night that covers me
Black as the pit from pole to pole
I thank whatever Gods there be
For my unconquerable soul.'

Q,2. COVID has become the new religion, a new movement which is replacing the old politics.

Q,3. Part of me at 71 is glad I won't see the destruction. The other part wants to know how everyone survives. I am so glad I am not raising my family now. I would be suffering from anxiety daily on their behalf.

A,2. I think that the virus and man-made global warming are indeed becoming an intertwined new religion. It seems to be the same true believers caught up in the fervor, and the same gauleiters issuing similar mandates. The obvious fear is that as, or if, the virus recedes, global warming will take over with similar lockdowns and restrictions.

February 10 at 1:47 PM

At the hospital today. The outpatient clinic almost empty as patients are too afraid to come to downtown Toronto. People are terrified of the subway, but buses are packed with so-called essential workers. Media has made people frightened of hospitals, in spite of screening which makes them much safer than the packed big box stores.

Looking at Canadian mortality figures. I know that at least 50% or many more reported deaths are with, not due to the virus. That is true for all countries. In the US it is probably closer to 90%. Death rates began to rise again in October, seem to have peaked in January, and are falling. This surprised me as I thought it would be the end of March or early April before the virus passed through and deaths would vanish as they did last year. Joe's 100 day masking would by then be over, testing could stop and the epidemic declared at an end.

The figures suggest that Canada was lightly hit last spring, leaving more vulnerable people or 'dry tinder' as some Europeans say. Perhaps this silly summer lockdown and the introduction of mandatory masking during the safe summer spread season, if it did anything at all, led to less community immunity and therefore more infections in early winter and therefore more deaths. Correlation doesn't equal causation but look at the graphs yourselves.

The utterly inexplicable public health recommendations continue. As R.W. Emerson wrote in 1856,

'Far and forgot to me is near,
Shadow and sunlight are the same.
The vanished gods to me appear
And one to me is shame and fame.'

Canada claims, based on the laughable inaccurate PCR testing, to be one of the most affected countries. And yet Ottawa has just banned cruise ships from entering Canadian waters, which makes absolutely no sense. So tourism in Alaska and the North East coast has gone for this year and probably the next. Cruise ships are probably one of the safer places and I would love to be on one right now, standing at the rail, in the sunshine, watching the sea slide by. But I fear on return to Canada our Dear Leader would insist on 2 weeks or more in one of his quarantine camps or hotels, even if you have a negative test. There is no logic to any of this. I suppose you have to be a government man to understand.

And schools, which are still not open in Ontario, will close in a few weeks for March break, because teachers are so stressed they need a holiday. I thought that it was appalling that kids, who were at no risk at all, missed a year off school. Someone just pointed out to me that school doesn't actually teach anything useful any more. Kids come out of 13 years of school knowing nothing, and much of what they have been told is not true, so they can't find a job. So maybe not going to school for a year is OK. The kids may be better off. Time will tell.

Q,1. I agree when it comes to school. We did more at home, and missed all the sex-ed classes, the 'spirit of the week', 'waste of time week' and so on. I pulled my daughter out of any political indoctrination class. Other than socializing, I am not terribly positive about the curriculum in our schools. When do we as a society push back?

A,1. My last son attended one of the supposedly most academic schools in Toronto. He was taught no history, nothing, except some totally irrelevant Canadian stuff. No Egypt, no Greece, no Rome, no Spain, no British, no American, nada! How can you understand the world if you know nothing about it? I hear kids can graduate from university arts courses without ever reading Shakespeare or Kit Marlowe. So I am inclined to agree, school ain't worth much.

February 12 at 5:06 PM

'Gaudeamus igitur, juvenes dum sumus,' 'Let us be happy while we are young.' We used to sing that when I was an undergraduate at St. Andrews university a long time ago, none too sober and seldom in tune. Last year, and it looks like this year, the young will not be allowed to be happy because of a disease which doesn't affect them. The most recent figures I can get still state that only one child under age 19 has died of the virus in all Canada.

The Public Health Johnnies (PHJs) continue to terrify the populace by claiming huge numbers of infected cases in the young, based on this completely unreliable test. They sound like Francis Bacon (1610) describing the fly, sitting on the axle tree of the chariot wheel, saying, 'what a dust I raise!' The PHJs certainly have raised a dust storm and blown it into the eyes of the politicians and media.

Clinic quiet today, so reading Santayana, who wrote, 'fanaticism consists of redoubling your effort when you have forgotten your aim.' The lockdown was supposed to flatten the curve, which it never did, in any country, and protect the hospitals, which were never in trouble, outside a very few in Italy, Spain and New York.

Listening this morning to some clever people discussing problems with the PCR test. One judge in Portugal has rejected it as a reliable indicator of disease. The original paper, on which the PCR test is based, which was rushed into publication last year, is now being challenged by numerous people as being essentially non diagnostic of disease, as the original developer, always said, especially when run at a multiplier of 37x or more.

Others were discussing social distancing. Some docs were saying there is actually no clinical evidence in human studies. It makes sense to avoid crowded events, but they point out that jam-packed big box stores, demonstrations and riots have not produced a spike in cases. So closing mom and pop stores makes no scientific or common sense. So why do it? Ockham's razor is that the simplest explanation is probably the correct one. So was it stupidity or cupidity? You choose.

We are now being told that this virus mutation, which has been about since September, is going to be deadly in April. I suppose, all things are possible. But for a seasonal virus which last year went away, then it is pretty unlikely. Mutations of clever viruses get more infectious and less deadly. Maybe this is different, but there is no data to suggest it is.

TS Elliot wrote, 'March is the cruelest month.' But the death rate in Canada is falling surprisingly rapidly. The days are getting longer, and maybe soon the vulnerable and the worried well can get the vaccine. I just hope it will not be forced on those who don't want it, and on children who don't need it.

Q,1. I am vulnerable because I don't have a spleen, but I am not so keen to have a vaccine. Is it safe?

A,1. I really don't know as there has been so little testing, and obviously no long term studies. Theoretically those with a less robust immune system are safer, as in them the vaccine is less likely to produce a hyperimmune response. But realistically, no one knows.

Q, 2. I know someone who works in health care, who told me that two elderly women who were in good health got the vaccine and died shortly after. There is no way I am taking that vaccine.

A,2. I didn't respond to that comment as it would have rendered this post liable to instant censorship, but I have heard the same thing. It is interesting to look at numerous country's death rates which skyrocketed when the vaccine was introduced. Correlation does not equal causation, but with the same results in country after country, it looks awfully convincing. I am waiting for more information or an explanation.

February 15 at 3:57 PM

Clinic quiet. A provincial holiday, in Canada, in February, freezing outside and a snow storm on the way, and everything in lockdown. Just who thinks this is a good time to have a holiday? In Florida the sun is shining and everything is open. I gave up my Florida medical license 10 years ago. Clearly having an advanced medical degree doesn't make you smart.

'Now is the winter of our discontent,' (Richard 111), made glorious by the CDC claiming that two masks are necessary, or maybe 3, or 4. As a surgeon I have worn a mask all my life. Checked the mortality figures. In Canada dropping like a stone. Zero deaths by virus in Ontario yesterday. Surprised, I thought it would be April before it went away. US figures are meaningless as they changed the definition last year, so they count any death with the virus as a death of the virus. Even there, the rate is flattening. So what's with the masking?

Universal masking was introduced last summer when there were virtually no deaths, immunity was at its height, people were outside, spaced and in the sunshine. It made absolutely no sense then. Was it to keep up the fear level? Is that what this cry for double masking is all about? Just asking.

Looking again at the Diamond Princess. A perfect experiment. Of the 1,000 crew, none died. Of the 3,000 passengers, 14 died, one under age 70. This, and the Swedish experience showed that universal lockdown was never indicated, or at least should have been lifted as soon as these figures were available, certainly by May of 2020.

Instead the West threw out all its accumulated knowledge and followed the Chinese communists. No one I know understands why. Clearly essentially no healthy person under 60 or 70 was at risk, and only the vulnerable required protection.

Listening to a clever doc discussing the theory of 'strain development'. If the pool of victims is reduced, the virus mutates to infect more susceptibles. So lockdown, if it had any effect at all, which no study has shown, by reducing the number exposed, stimulated the virus to mutate. That makes sense.

The response of the Western world has been inexplicable. If they were really worried about a second wave, then use the summer when hospitals were empty to build more capacity and cross train more ICU staff. But the new built military hospitals, which were essentially never used, were taken down.

Even WHO now claims that there is no place for lockdown. So why continue? Any ideas?

Q,1. Maybe we should go with Ockham's razor conclusion: the Chinese created a bioweapon which catastrophically disrupted international commerce and incarcerated formerly free peoples throughout the world.

Q,2. The involvement of American and international organizations in the Wuhan lab project is an open secret. Again, the obvious question, cui bono?

Q,3. It is necessary to keep everyone afraid of the virus so they can sell all these vaccines. If it is no longer a big deal, no one will get the vaccine.

Q,4. The lockdowns have become a political tool. In dictatorships the supreme leaders like Xi have images to worship everywhere. In Canada we have no sitting parliament but our supreme leader gets TV time every day. We will go from a pandemic to climate change and the politics of fear will continue.

A,1. All of these comments make sense. That was what I was afraid of. The virus fear will transition smoothly into the fear of global warming. And so the farce continues. Was this the original purpose?

February 18 at 9:28 PM

I have collected all my posts from last year and have published them in book form. It is now available on Amazon. I would like to thank all those whose thoughtful comments, questions, and observations I have edited and added. I was just in time, as some of the posts have been removed, including the one where I described and admired the lace face mask I saw in a ladies lingerie store window.

I really took no interest in the Wuhan virus until March, as there are always panics about something, like H1N1, global warming, Ebola, thinning of the ozone layer, MERS, running out of oil, etc. But then it seemed like this was The Big One, with a 3% mortality, a huge death rate. I thought all of us medical people would die. But then Charite in Berlin suggested 0.3%, still huge but manageable. Then we heard the Bat Lady had added HIV, stolen from the lab in Winnipeg, which would mean no immunity. It was May before the Koreans showed that 20% were late excreters, and that if Bat Woman had added HIV, it was inactive. All the docs in the world rejoiced as this meant that there was immunity.

I found I was answering so many questions in the clinic and on Facebook that what I was doing was creating a Journal of a Plague Year. So I thought about publishing, as so many great scientists and docs were being silenced. The original Journal of the Plague Year was written by Daniel Defoe in 1665.

And then came spring and death rates almost vanished, as you would expect with a seasonal virus. The fear was kept going with this PCR test run at 37x on people with no symptoms. And this inexplicable mandatory masking. No preparations at all were made for a winter resurgence.

Reviewing the world data, death rates are dropping rapidly, a month earlier than I expected. The Public Health Johnnies keep trying to frighten the people with double masking and a mutant virus. They seem unwilling or unable to understand that a virus mutates to infect more people and kill less. The UK figures, where the mutant has been flourishing for months, are like Canada, dropping rapidly, so hopefully the real epidemic, as opposed to the Casedemic, will be over soon.

The world's inexplicable reaction to this virus is such that I continue to collect posts in case the reaction continues for another Plague Year (2021).

Q,1. Thank you for publishing your posts. How shocking that the media colluded to suppress critical information. They allow the oligopoly which governs us to operate in secret.

Q,2. We have to try to expose this Plandemic by sharing information which the legacy media is suppressing.

A,1. For a short time my book seemed to have vanished from Amazon. I thought it had been censored, but then it came back. It is frightening that I thought that that had actually happened, in North America. Self-censorship is required to avoid being deplatformed. A decade ago who would ever have thought of very careful self-censorship before putting pen to paper, or that any written article or book written in the West, could be censored?

February 23 at 12:20 PM

Great sense of relief! My new book, Journal of the Plague Year (2020), which many of you helped me to write, is now back on Amazon and all the other book sellers. When it disappeared I thought I had hit a land mine and would be gone. But I guess I get to live another day.

In the middle of all this chaos, some things make life livable. Came out of the clinic to go home. I was getting into the car when a guy pointed out a flat tire. Sinking feeling. I haven't changed a tire in 20 years. Called CAA and found I had forgotten to renew. Girl on the phone renewed it in 3 minutes, giving me a large discount. Truck turned up in 5 minutes. Tyre reinflated, drove home to my usual garage at the end of the street. They found a nail in the tire and fixed it immediately. All so smooth and so efficient. If it had been the government, I would still be waiting in the parking lot. And yesterday, driving on the 401 highway, 24 lanes of traffic, in heavy snow, smooth and fast. We humans are pretty good if left alone.

News of the virus is still leaking. Canadian soldiers who competed in the Military games in Wuhan in the fall of 2019 came home sick with a respiratory infection. That knowledge was covered up. I have lectured and operated in China for many years. The first time was more than thirty years ago. Their medical system is hospital based. To be treated you need to go to hospital. If you are not admitted you basically don't get treated. So if you are sick and sent home and die, you are not a virus death. And the three companies, designated to produce the tests. Look it up yourself. I am afraid - - - - -.(Now I feel safe to tell you. They had connections with the CCP and had no prior experience in this field, so the tests were as accurate or as inaccurate as you would expect. What is so odd was that I felt if I mentioned the connection to the CCP I would have been immediately censored.)

When I was a student, I wanted to build bridges, not be a philosopher or psychologist. The docs who taught me psychiatry, thought psychologists were charlatans, and that mental diseases were undiscovered brain diseases. Like stomach ulcers, as when I was a student those needed surgery. Now you take some pills for a week.

But I could not understand the unimaginable response to this tightly targeted virus, which really affected only the ill elderly. Yes, yes! I know lots of money was made by friends of friends, and there were huge political gains. But why did almost the whole world accept house arrest?

Thousands of docs, engineers and scientists had to have known, at least since the end of May, that lockdown, masking, social distancing, and the rest, had no basis in science and were damaging beyond all belief. I despaired as William Tell, John Huss, and Martin Luther were missing. 'Here I stand. I can do none other. God help me.'

I found that these people actually were there, but they were being silenced. And tragically there was no outcry over their silencing.

Who ever thought I would listen to Carl Jung? But he describes what is happening. He calls it 'animus possessed', that people have been infected by an irrational belief. Like wearing a mask on your own in your car.

Jung and especially Nietzsche thought that the moral ideals of Western civilization were collapsing. Most people need to believe in something. If they stopped believing in God, which many obviously have, as seen by the desperate edicts of the lockdownists to keep churches closed, then they will worship the state, which by definition is totalitarianism.

In the face of falling death rates, the PHJs still strive to terrify the populace with threats of 3rd or 4th waves. They ignore that the virus mutant has been in the UK since the fall, and death rates there have been falling since January, just like Canada. I guess they missed the lecture in medical school when it was explained that a clever virus mutates to infect more people and kill less.

Q,1. Reading about John Huss and Martin Luther in The Great Controversy. Again, for the first time in twenty years. In love with both of them, and many others.

A,1. Today we sure need these heroes of old.

Q,2. I believe the virus was purposely set loose for several reasons. Mainly to change leaders and ensure the new world order, and secondly for money. God help us all.

A,2. Indeed, God help us all. Pray for us now in the hour of our darkness.

February 25 at 3:42 PM

Funny, the older I get the more I like Latin. 'Iam seges est ubi Troia fuit.' 'There is now a cornfield where Troy once stood.' (Ovid, AD 10). The topless towers of Ilium (Troy) have fallen, and Balkh, the mother of cities, lies in ruins. How quickly it can all fall apart. The British Empire collapsed in 40 years and the Soviet in 10.

The churches in the US have been closed by politicians, and people just accept it. Gerard de Nerval (1845), 'Dieu est mort! Le ciel est vide. Pleurez enfants, vous n'avez plus de pere.' 'God is dead! Weep children, you no longer have a father.'

Maybe all is not lost, but when I look at the passive subservience of the bulk of the population to incompetent, untrustworthy politicians - -'thank you master for locking us up.'

I am a Cameron and our clan motto was, 'touch not the cat without a glove.' If any child dared to say such a thing today, he would be immediately diagnosed as 'toxic masculinity,' or an 'Attention Deficit Disorder' and drugged with Ritalin.

In the face of all scientific evidence, lockdown continues in Canada. The PHJs continue to bleat about a 3rd wave, completely ignoring the mortality statistics, showing plunging death rates in the UK where the virus mutant has been in action since September. The whole theory of lockdown was anti-scientific to begin with and was completely destroyed by Sweden and Florida. So why does it persist? Why are the little guy's stores closed, and the big box stores jammed with people?

And quarantine! The concept was developed in Venice to keep out the plague. Ships had to remain outside the city for quaranta giorni, 40 days. It is to keep the disease out. Once it is in, quarantine serves no purpose.

Obviously it makes sense for protective quarantine of the susceptible, once you know who they are, like care homes.

Is there light at the end of the tunnel, or is this the Gotterdammerung, the twilight of the West? The original Pope Benedict said, 'pruned it grows again.' But Augustine, the Bishop of Hippo, watching from North Africa the lights go out in Rome, said, 'it is finished.' And it was. The lights remained out for 1,000 years.

I hope not! I really hope not. It all seemed so different when I first came to Canada. 'In the glad morning of our days.' We would so like to be able to say to the next generation, as Dr John McCrae wrote in the devastation of WW1,

'to you we fling the torch,
be yours to hold it high.'

But I fear the light has gone out and the darkness comes again.

It must be the Canadian winter depression. I need to go to Florida.

Q,1. Yours is a common sensation, one of hopelessness and some defiance. More need to say 'enough' and get on with life. Real life, not one constricted by government babysitting and regulations. It is obvious that the pioneer spirit that built our country is missing. The common comparison to sheep is a viable one. We are like these animals, led and herded into pens, totally dependent on the masters. Time to come to life and be the strong citizens we once were.

Q,2. California is opening back up now. Our church has been holding outside services since October. We will go back inside next Sunday. Can't wait!!

Q,3. In the Phoenix area our church has been open since May 2020. We have two services and we spread out. Our church suggests masks but does not enforce it.

Q,4. In Florida I've seen Americans going on with their normal lives. Here I'm afraid to go for my morning walks and coffee. (This lady is seriously immunocompromised, so her fear is justified.)

Q,4. April Fool's Day has been canceled this year. Because no prank is greater than the joke that is running Canada right now.

A,1. What can you say? All these comments are absolutely valid. It is nice to see that Americans have not forgotten God.

March 1 at 6:30 PM

Soren Kierkegaard 1850 wrote that 'life can only be understood backwards, but must be lived forwards.' Looking back at the events of the inexplicable year, as I have outlined in my new book 'Journal of the Plague Year (2020)', I think that he is correct.

Immanuel Kant wrote that truth will eventually reveal itself. He may have been right about many things, but he was plain wrong on that. Truth can be buried so deeply that by the time it trickles out, if ever, no one cares. Like the lies written by the New York Times reporter, Walter Duranty, about the glorious Soviet, and that good guy, Joe Stalin. Did they ever ask that 'fellow traveler' to give back his Pulitzer Prize?

My children in Toronto were taught no history, none at all, which I think is now standard in the Anglo world. They know nothing of the glories of Greece, Rome, or Spain. All around the Anglo world I see history being erased, even the events of the last decade. With so many being silenced, what will be the eventual official history of the Great Virus Caper?

This virus episode has precedents in history, like the 'Great Leap Forwards' in China, otherwise known as 'The Great Starvation,' and the Cultural Revolution, which I suppose is fitting as they come from the same place as the virus. It still continues with misinformation being trumped by the media and the PHJs, and teachers unions. Why they continue is not clear.

All you need to do is google COVID deaths and then the country, like the UK. Don't look at the so-called cases, as these are simply positive tests which usually mean nothing. In most Northern countries, the winter resurgence peaked in January and is falling rapidly. Sweden, the country that the PHJs insist they have never heard of, is doing very well, with no masking, lockdown or much of anything else.

Will the availability of the vaccination end the world wide panic? Well maybe, but why did it start in the first place? Does the CDC continue to fund work in the virology lab in Wuhan? Are they still working on 'gain of function' to make the next virus more effective? Universal masking was brought in last summer when there were virtually no deaths, and now I am told even after the vaccine it will be necessary to wear 2 or 3 masks for how long? Forever?

The small businesses have been ruined by lockdown. The global warmists seem to be back in action to ruin what is left of manufacturing, by driving up energy costs. I had hoped that with the computer modelers having been obviously so utterly and repeatedly wrong with something as simple as a virus, that no one would believe them when they talked about climate.

Oh well, spring is coming. But with the Grand Solar Minimum in full swing it is likely to be slow and cold. I hope not.

Q,1. In answer to your question, does the CDC still fund the work in the Wuhan lab? I ran across this article which shows that the US Feds have just authorized funding for the Wuhan lab until January 2024. (She gave the website.)

Q,2. The Soviets rewrote their history, so I am sure the current governments will try. I have to wonder how our children will remember it.

A,1. Given the current attempts to rewrite history in the US, who knows what will be told of the Great Virus Scam. State education, at least in the Anglo world, teaches no history. In China children are still taught, or used to be, that Mao was a great leader who loved his people.

March 6 at 3:00 PM

Just spent the last 90 minutes listening to what happened in China with the virus. The time lines may be accurate enough, but the facts are clearly in doubt. There are far more questions than answers. Was this a false flag operation start to finish? Was it a culling? The virus was, after all, tightly targeted at the ill elderly, the unproductive on CCP government pensions.

It sounds like a vast conspiracy, as Kipling wrote, 'truths, twisted by knaves to make a trap for fools.' But experience with governments, universities, and big business is that their mistakes are usually due to incompetence rather than malevolence. Although, given the ease with which truth can be vanished, this could certainly enable a series of conspiracies, acting in parallel.

Universal lockdown had no basis in science. Sweden destroyed that theory. Lockdown completely failed to protect the vulnerable and actually exposed them more. In all countries the essential workers, the poor, the cleaners, truck drivers, were exempted from lockdown. There was no spike in disease in grocery store clerks, who initially had no masks, no distancing, and no shields. So why does lockdown continue?

This fiasco has been called the biggest medical mistake the world has ever seen. Masking is a fig leaf and people are impervious to data. Joseph Schumpeter said that 'workers would produce enough money to produce a parasitic class who produce nothing and would attack them'. Is this really what is happening with the destruction of mom and pop stores, and the coming destruction of industry in the West by the Global Warmists closing pipelines?

In Rome and Athens we look at the ruins of great civilizations, and even in Paris, a roofless Notre Dame. So civilizations do collapse. Kipling wrote,

'low among the alders lie the derelict foundations,
the beams whereon they trusted
and the plinths whereon they built.
My rulers and their treasures and their unborn
generations, dead, destroyed - -'

Nietzsche predicted that the collapse of the moral ideals of the West would be followed by nihilism or by worship of the state, totalitarianism. That certainly seems to be happening. Today we are also seeing the death of science and it's replacement by Scientism. Alternate views are suppressed as heresy. The weasel words are 'denier' used by the cancel culture. It is like Orwell's 1984, 'follow the science', or '90% of scientists agree,' which means exactly the opposite.

It is all too gloomy to contemplate. At least the days are getting longer, but as we are entering a grand solar minimum, it is likely to be a long cold spring. This last year has made us conscious, as someone said, that 'we may live in the shadow of death, but we should try to live in the light of Life.'

Q,1. Too true. I am still astonished by the total complacency and accommodation of the populace when given strange and conflicting decrees by government. The acceptance, immediate and unquestioning is frightening in its import for the future. The powerful, be they elected or wealthy, have found themselves in total control for the most part of the little people like you and me. The future is clouded and it looks increasingly like 1984.

Q,2. So painfully true and frightening. We can see the apocalypse coming, and there is no organized defense against it.

Q,3. How WHO faked the pandemic. Read an article from Forbes in 2010. This was in response to the H1N1 scam of 2009. The same players tried the same tactics. Then they failed. This time they succeeded. (Reference given.)

A,1. I knew that WHO had changed the definition of an epidemic and pandemic removing the word 'lethal', fatal, or deadly. This means that any winter outbreak of flu can be called an epidemic and politicians can bring in a lockdown any winter, or if an unreliable and easily manipulated test like the PCR is used, anytime, anywhere,

Q,4. Same script, same tactics, same players. 10 years ago they tried the same thing.

A,4. Plus ça change, plus c'est la même chose. They tried it with bird flu, H1N1 and finally succeeded with this virus.

Q,5. Karl Marx thought using science and technology to push a socialist agenda was a good idea.

A,5. Yes, and look where the socialist agenda ended up, The Red Terror, The Killing Fields, The Holodomor, The Great Hunger, and on and on.

March 9 at 4:44 PM

No clinic today so walking in the sunshine. Only March, so the Canadian winter is not over. Almost Sakura time in Japan, but no visits this year as the ruler of Canada and his PHJs have decided to forcibly quarantine anyone who dares to leave and return.

One brave returning nurse told the quarantine camp guards and officials at the Toronto airport to get lost and walked out. Many in Canada cheered her bravado, but sadly, not all. A percentage of the population have come to like absolute government control of their lives.

Interestingly, in one short stretch of road, there were 3 Pot shops and one liquor store. They were open while almost everything else was closed. Was Huxley actually correct in his book The Brave New World? Has the great reset actually taken place. With restaurants and stores closed, all it takes is to prevent schools from opening and then there's no reason to leave home. The net for home entertainment, and food and recreational drugs delivered to your door.

The few people on the street mostly were widely distanced and wearing masks. Surely by now most people know that masks are worthless. They don't prevent the wearer from infection and if wet, reused or touched they actually spread infection, if there is any. In Japan or Korea if you have a cold you wear a mask, but single use and change frequently. If you have no symptoms, are alone and in the sunshine, just what is a mask supposed to do?

In most northern countries the virus death rates continue to plummet. It is still not clear what constitutes a virus death, and almost certainly at least 50% can be discounted. The deaths peaked in January, which surprised me, as I thought it would be February or March. But it looks like the winter resurgence is over. But I suppose that the media and PHJs will continue to spread panic until they can use up all these vaccinations they have purchased at great expense.

We look around at the wreckage and ask why? Why did the West abandon all its collective medical knowledge? Why did Sweden alone follow the standard teachings? WHO, following their Chinese master's orders, was obviously one of the main drivers, but a study of the net shows that they have tried that in the past also, just not successfully. They tried it with H1N1, and other flu outbreaks. But this time many countries listened to and followed the Pied Piper. Why?

In many countries it was obviously purely political, and perhaps in others purely financial. It is just hard for any rational person to believe that they would do this for money and power. The deaths from lockdown due to despair, with suicide, alcohol and drugs are not reported. Similarly no one knows what the deaths from untreated cancer, heart disease and strokes have been and will be. We hear rumors of millions but have no figures on the starvations to come. With the global warmists again trying to destroy cheap energy, the famines to come are likely to make the horrors of the Holodomor and the Great Leap Forward (the Great Hunger) look like a walk in the park. Surely this was not what it was all about?

Q,1. So many are simply speaking sheep, going along with everything.

A,1. It is sad. Where is the young 'roaring boy's bravado'? Instead it is left to a single bold, beautiful, brassy lass to tell the airport quarantine goons to buzz off.

Q,2. I don't know how to respond other than to point out that so many have become conditioned and so many believe lies. There is hardly any critical thinking, no skepticism, and no thoughtful logic. There is no simple wondering if we are being played by politicians.

Q,3. My own doctor has said the same thing, that people are not getting the care they need because of fear. He said that there will be far more non virus deaths.

Q,4. This is only the beginning. Look at the interconnected power grids and how easily they are hacked and shut down. And yet we are expected to go from gas powered transportation to electric. What happens when a grid is shut down? Where in the world is there critical thinking?

A,2. There were many more thoughtful comments like this. What more is there to say? I agree with them all. Why is none of this discussed in the halls of the academe or by the legacy media?

March 14 at 6:27 PM

'Oh judgment, thou art fled to brutish beasts, and men have lost their reason.' So said Mark Anthony, mourning Caesar, but a fitting epitaph of the ongoing lunacy.

Just thinking, was the world always so crazy? Maybe it was. Look at the South Sea Bubble, the Great Leap Forwards, the New Deal, the mortgage delusion, global warming, the Tulip mania, etc.

The horrors of the Soviet Union and Mao's China were covered up for years by the legacy media. It wasn't as if the truth was unknown. The media simply ignored it. Even today, when everyone knows about the 100 million corpses, one still hears university people and others declare that they are Marxists. If they actually know anything about Marxism and its results they should be ashamed. Is this ignorance or malevolence?

I hear Dr Seuss has been banned for reasons I don't understand. I would strongly suggest everyone buy a copy of Alice in Wonderland, because it is sure to be next. The Social Justice Warriors are bound to find something with which they disagree. Although maybe not, as they all sound like the Red Queen. When Alice tells her she can't believe in the impossible, the Red Queen tells her to grow up. 'When I was your age, I could believe in as many as six impossible things before breakfast.' Just like a SJW.

Maybe we should list some of the impossible things the media expects us to believe.

Quarantine camps/ hotels. You have to get a negative test to get on a plane to Canada, but they will still insist on arrival you quarantine in their camps at your own expense. Clearly the PHJs missed the lecture on quarantine at medical school. Once a disease is inside a country quarantine serves no purpose.

Universal masking in the middle of summer when there were virtually no deaths. Actually universal masking at any time is simply silly.

The PCR test run at 37x. The man who developed the test said this was wrong. It detects a bit of a dead virus, possibly a corona, but doesn't mean anyone is ill. Yesterday in Ontario there were 1,700 positive tests and 15 deaths. This is called a Casedemic, as seen last summer. This means you have cases, but no actual illnesses.

You need the vaccine after you have had the disease! This is contrary to all medical teaching. Until May last year, when the Koreans showed that everyone had immunity post infection, we were terrified that Bat Woman had added HIV stolen from the Winnipeg lab. I describe in my book Journal of the Plague Year (2020) the enormous sense of relief, when we found that immunity to the Wuhan virus existed. If the HIV component was active there would be no immunity.

One could go on and on; the closing of mom and pop stores, beauticians, gyms, and then encouraging demonstrations and riots and jamming into big box stores.

In some ways, the worst of all, keeping kids out of school. They have lost a year, a year they will never get back. And yet we knew by May of 2020 that this was completely unnecessary. It could be worse I suppose. It is spring, and as the Rubaiyat says,

'Come fill the cup and in the fire of spring
The winter garment of repentance fling
The bird of time has but a little way to fly
And lo, the bird is on the wing.'

Q,1. I live in a small, isolated community. We had a bad outbreak last year and lost a lot of people in the large nursing home. The staff were in and out of small businesses here, grocery stores, convenience stores, etc. yet there was no community outbreak. By May 2020 the outbreak was finally over inside the nursing home. During this time there was no community spread. How could we have avoided this if it were as contagious as the government is trying to convince us? I am just an ordinary person with an ordinary mind. But if I can see this, why can't others? The government scaremongering continues a year later and still people are scared to death.

A,1. What you are describing is most people's experience. We knew by May 2020, that this was not 'The Big One'. Inexplicably the government continues to act as if it was.

Q,2. My mother-in-law is a physical train wreck; you name it she has it. She got the virus, recovered after convalescent plasma, and is as mean as ever.

A,2. We all have these little crosses to bear. Thank modern medicine.

Q,3. The looking glass is broken. We live in a world of make believe and fools.

A,3. It looks that way when you see people wearing a dirty, wet, reused mask outside. When they crowd into big box stores and buses and the tiny mom and pop stores are closed by government mandate.

March 18 at 5:54 PM

Listening to a Public Health Johnny (PHJ) on the car radio on the way to work. Depressingly unintelligent. Talleyrand (1814) described them. 'They have learned nothing and forgotten nothing.' While checking that he actually said that and not Fouche', as I always mix up these two guys, I found another of his quotes. 'Society is divided into the shearers and the shorn.' For the last year most of us have been the shorn.

This PHJ was wailing on about the need for further lockdown in Ontario, one of the world's most lockdown sub countries. We are being overwhelmed by the new mutant virus. Two weeks of serious lockdown would be the cure!! I know PHJs are not the sharpest nails in the box, but how can one be wrong in so many ways at once?

They continue to base all their models on this near to useless PCR test run at a 37x multiplier. A positive test means virtually nothing; certainly not a sick person or one who transmits. Simply look at the death rate. In Ontario in the middle of the Canadian winter only 15 people died yesterday with no information on age or comorbidities. So how many actually died of the virus? 5? 10? And for this more lockdown?

And this failure to understand that a clever virus mutates to infect more people and kill less. The data from England shows the death rate plummeting since January, in spite of the new mutant virus being there since September.

And two weeks to flatten the curve! Carl Jung would describe these people as 'animus possessed,' full of irrational ideas. I guess these people never heard of Florida, which did everything right in terms of virus management.

The clinic today was full of kids; fat, depressed, with sore backs. How could they not be? They have been in house arrest for a year, for a disease which never affected them. Even the sainted Dr. has just admitted that there never was any reason to close schools. He has also just admitted that social distancing was a fantasy. Now if he would only admit that universal masking is silly. The way it is done it spreads disease, not limit it.

I feel so sorry for these poor kids. They need to go back to school with no masks, no distancing, no restrictions. The boys I would like to go to basketball and the girls to dance classes. The coaches and instructors are very tough. They teach the kids poise, respect, and discipline. All their aches and pains go away. And get them out into the sunshine.

I have been taking copies of my new book Journal of the Plague Year (2020), to the clinic and interestingly they have been selling out. I guess people no longer believe anything from the legacy media and would like to know what is actually happening. They don't know who to trust, and how would they? I could suggest names, but so many excellent docs and scientists have been canceled by social media. I am afraid to do so in case I am canceled for naming them. How could the West reach this state?

People are beginning to wake up and realize that what they are being told makes no sense. They can't go to a mom and pop store but can jam into a big box store. They can't go to a restaurant with healthy friends but can jam into a city bus with coughing strangers. But how do you rebel? Yesterday I was forced to sit an Equity and Inclusion exam in order for my annual reappointment at the hospital. What this has to do with medicine I have no idea but am afraid it will get worse.

Oh well, summer is coming!

Q,1. It is truly sad what the globalists have reduced the world to in one short year. Keep the faith good sir, for there truly is strength in numbers, and the longer this goes on the larger our numbered will become

A,1. Deus Vult. God willing!

March 22 at 5:09 PM

Just when one thinks that there is light at the end of this nightmare of last year, the Canadian media is full of terror of a third wave of a mutant virus. 1,700 new cases in Ontario. But of course they are not cases. They are positive PCR tests, which are essentially meaningless. Surely even the dullest media person can google virus death rates in any country. There were 33 deaths in all Canada yesterday, with of course no details on age and comorbidities.

The dreaded English version, loose since September, killed 33 in the UK yesterday. And we are supposed to be scared of this?

Was it ever thus? When did most of us realize that truth and the Legacy media have little connection? Presumably they work on the principle that half the populace will believe anything they are told, and they can write off the other half. They seem utterly oblivious to the harm they are doing to the children. Maybe that's how a culture ends. If the children don't matter, then nothing else does.

The so-called education in the West has been abysmal for decades. I remember the shock and despair I felt when I found that my last son knew no history, none at all. Canada is an immigrant country, and so many know the wonderful history of their own peoples, the glories of Persia, Greece, Rome, Spain, and Britain. If you don't know history you know nothing.

And literature - in the school which is supposed to be the most academic in Canada - my son was asked to review Macbeth through a Marxist lens. I wish I was making that up. I hear things are equally bad in the US. In Canada the kids have never heard of Vimy Ridge, and in the US of Lexington and Valley Forge. Tragically so few even know the moving lyrics of The Battle Hymn of the Republic-

'as he died to make men holy
let us live to make men free.'

What more magnificent lines are there in all the world? We used to sing that in my father's church in a tiny mining village in Scotland. 'Let the hero born of woman crush the serpent with his heel.'

But so it goes. As Newbolt wrote,

'There's a far bell ringing at the setting of the sun,
and a phantom voice is singing of the great days done.'

If you can bear to listen to the ineffable unfolding tragedy, just google the video of the Soviet defector. In 1984 he described exactly what would happen and it has. The Long March through education, entertainment, and politics is almost complete. Even the STEM fields are failing. Look at how few new patents there are, less every year as universities fill up with quotas of 'has beens' and 'never wasses'.

And the PHJs, who can't read a Gompertz curve, and have never heard of Sweden and Florida, or of death rates. Their mishandling of this virus is going to be the greatest medical disaster in the world's history. But why, was it malevolence or stupidity? In sober moments they surely must feel like Faust. Will they ever regret the damage they have done to the young? Faust sold his soul to the devil. Kit Marlowe (1590) 'that Faustus may repent and save his soul.' He may have repented, but the Devil took him anyway.

Q,1. Yuri Bezmenov knew it and it started in the US in the 1930s and was institutionalized in our Department of 'Education' which came into existence in 1980. People don't see what is happening because they have deliberately been kept ignorant of history, and too few parents fill in the gap. But I remain hopeful that eventually good will triumph over evil.

Q,2. Maybe I am crazy, but this looks planned. Klaus of Davos doesn't even try to conceal that this virus is his great chance for The Great Reset.

Q,3. I noticed history was being wiped out of education. But what have they replaced it with?

Q,4. It's a sad day, and it's going to get even sadder yet.

A,1. Everything that these readers have said is true. How will this end? Will it ever be possible to reintroduce History and Civics into state education in the West? Without knowledge of the past, how can you have any idea about the future? Is this truly a planned event?

March 25 at 3:50 PM

Almost spring! Friends in Japan posting photos of Sakura, cherry blossoms. It symbolizes the fleeting beauty of life. As Robert Burns wrote

'Like the snowfall in the river
one moment white, then gone forever,
Or like the Borealis race
That flits ere you can point the place.
Or like the rainbow's lovely form
Evanishing amid the storm.'

Even in Canada, the coldest country in the world. Kipling wrote,

'Robin down the logging road whistles come to me.
Spring has found the maple grove, the sap is running free.
All the winds of Canada call the plowing rain.'

Driving to work on the 401 highway. 24 packed lanes of traffic, fast and smooth. A miracle it is not carnage. We humans are pretty remarkable. Turned on the car radio. Wish I had not. A huge deficit budget. Another level of government thinks that they have found the magic money tree. I hate to rain on anyone's parade, but the Canadian dollar is not a reserve currency. If you want to see what it is actually worth, see what it costs in a grocery store, as almost all our food is imported. Hard to imagine, but will the 'great hunger' occur in Canada? The UN claims millions will face starvation as a result of the lockdown, not the virus.

And the depressing PHJs with their pathetic cries of woe. They have just admitted that the PCR test is being run at a 37x multiplier, and higher if nothing is found, so of course the numbers are going up. The tragedy is that the people making these statements must know that these claims have little to do with reality. ICU beds are almost full! But of course they are. They are so expensive that if they are not full they are closed. 4,000 positive tests yesterday in Canada but only 24 deaths, with as usual no data on age and comorbidities. A classic Casedemic!!

In Toronto you can have a massage but the beauty salons are closed. The PHJs clearly have no idea that only OR nurses and beauty salon staff are trained to avoid touching their face. Nails girls use gloves and shields, which makes them safer than any store and yet they are closed. And somehow this makes sense?

The only good news is that the PHJs are suggesting that if you have had the virus only one vac. is required. For centuries it has been taught that if you have had the disease you are immune. There are some exceptions, like amoebic dysentery. But suddenly in 2020 this knowledge disappeared. Like the Law of Gravity being repealed. There are downsides to excess immunity, so be thankful for small mercies, one jab only for your government travel permit. (Sadly, that ray of commonsense did not last long.)

The handling of this plague never made any sense. All medical knowledge was tossed away. Why?? Some of my earlier posts questioning this have disappeared, so I am glad I published the book before they all went. Google Journal of the Plague Year (2020). If you don't add 2020 you get Daniel Defoe's book published in 1722, about the Black Death which killed one third of Europe. It is quite instructive to see how they handled it.

I am still looking for excess deaths data. How much worse was it last year from previous years, or was it?

Q,1. Yes, food prices have gone up. What used to cost me at the store has tripled. Those on a fixed income will be hurt.

Q,2. Time to teach our kids how to grow food in the backyard.

A,1. Food prices are the best indication of what the Canadian dollar is worth, and it seems to be dropping rapidly.

Q,3. I hope travel permits will never be introduced into the US. Our HIPAA laws should prevent that.

A,3. I hope you are correct. But today I saw a couple playing tennis on an outdoor court where there was no one else. Both were wearing surgical face masks. I think people like that would welcome a vaccination passport.

March 30 at 6:24 PM

Good news/ bad news. Good news, in Toronto in March, no snow and the sun is shining. Medical clinic this morning is full of patients afraid to go to hospitals as the media has scared them. Hospitals are actually safer than big box stores. Selling out the first printing of my new book 'Journal of the Plague Year (2020)' as no one believes anything the legacy media tells them, and people want to know.

Bad news, the Public Health Johnnies (PHJs) and the media doomsayers as bad as ever. The sainted Dr now claims a new mutant can infect you without you knowing it and you can transmit it, and there is no test. So lockdown forever and wear 3 masks. Think about this new invisible disease! And you thought Alice in Wonderland was a kid's book. I guess 'shame' and 'responsible' are words which have been canceled.

And did you see the team WHO sent to Wuhan to investigate? 3 or 4 of the 'investigators' had working or financial relations with the Wuhan people. With a straight face, they claimed the virus came from imported frozen fish. Who knew that fish particles could float over the whole world?

The 'Terror' in Canada continues. The numbers are going up, so more lockdowns are coming. In spite of the fact that more than 20 scientific papers have been published showing lockdown has no positive effects, other than in small, isolated islands. In addition to the collateral deaths and economic damage, it is now suggested that lockdowns encourage mutants.

I looked up the figures and wept. In Alberta, a province being bankrupted by the central government's refusal to build pipelines, so we have to buy Middle East oil, yesterday there were 12,000 tests at around $140 per test. There were 550 positive tests and no deaths, zero deaths! A classic Casedemic. In the whole of Canada 110,000 tests and 17 deaths.

More people probably died falling down stairs, and certainly more of drug overdose. And the fentanyl also comes from Wuhan. In the whole UK, 23 died.

The net is full of tragic photos of kids wearing masks. As a surgeon I have worn a mask for 50 years. I can reassure parents that a loosely fitting surgical mask will not interfere with a child's breathing. (That was what I thought then, but there is new data which suggests that little children's CO2 levels may actually get too high while wearing a mask.) It does likely make them more liable to infection. I am not a psychologist, but I think the real problem for kids is going to be psychological. They can't see each other's faces, so they don't know how to read them, and they are taught that others carry a deadly disease. How can this fail to interfere with their socialization? All for a disease which we have known since last spring does not affect kids and they don't transmit. And the teachers, fighting desperately to keep schools closed, when they know that they are not at any risk. A shameful display. Clearly public education needs significant rethinking.

I found myself thinking and writing about this in my series of novels, 'To Slip the Surly Bonds of Earth.' The current education system is a disaster for the kids at the academic top and especially the bottom. Their needs are being completely ignored.

Addendum.

I have just learned that some face masks have been coated with graphene nanoparticles, supposedly to keep out a virus. But you can inhale these particles. I am told that they were sold in the province of Quebec only and have been withdrawn. As far as I know there is no graphene in regular surgical face masks.

Q,1. I guess old panties make a better mask.

A,1. Certainly a safer one. Since it is for show only, as masking is totally nonfunctional, I personally prefer old lace which has been washed repeatedly.

Q,2. 14 people died yesterday in Ontario and for this we are going into another lockdown. No word on age and comorbidities. And this makes sense to someone?

Q,3. Big pharma is certainly benefitting, and who else.

A,2. Cui Bono? as Cicero said in 50 BC. Who benefits?'

Q,4. It seems all facets of life have turned political. Some people have taken to stirring the vile pot of fear mongering to pit us against each other. We need to step up and stand out for freedoms which are being taken away from us.

A,4. I was in Braunschweig lecturing the night the East Germans said 'enough 'and tore down the wall. When will we say 'enough'?

April 4 at 7:00 PM

Holiday Sunday, the sun is shining, and the medical clinic is empty. Listening to Elon Musk. He was asked when A.I. (artificial intelligence), will turn us into cyborgs, part human/ part A.I. He pointed to his phone, "We are already." And he is right.

I never wanted a cellphone, but one US company I consult for eventually insisted. My son gave me his. I had no idea; it was magic, a whole new World. Any topic, anywhere, anytime. Philosophy in 5 minutes. I realized immediately, except for STEM, (the hard sciences), that universities were completely obsolete. Who needs to sit in a class and listen to some none-too-bright lecturer try to explain von Mises, when on my phone I can listen to the towering intellect of Tom Woods? Or works of Art, when I can listen to Roger Scruton, who is dead.

In retrospect, I already knew that universities were obsolete. In the 70s we were developing artificial hip and knee joints that actually worked. To sell them we had to teach surgeons how to put them in. A group of orthopedic surgeons, friends, and fierce competitors, traveled the world for 30 years, teaching and demonstrating surgery. We called ourselves the Traveling Road show. I wrote about the fun and frolics in my book 'Have Knife Will Travel'. In the West we bypassed universities, recognizing that their teaching model was obsolete.

And now the anti-science, hysterical response to the virus with the closing of schools and universities has demonstrated just how obsolete that medieval model actually is. My son, in engineering school, could be listening online from Kyoto, enjoying Sakura time, rather than sitting in London Ontario, enjoying what? The university experience? And who knows where his online lecturer physically is? Florida if he has any sense.

So what are the kids paying for? It is all online. So why not get a job, so there is no debt, and take courses in the evening? We surgeons, no matter where we train, all travel to one national central location to sit the same exam. That works perfectly well.

The response to this virus has shown appalling disregard for the poor children, as we have known since last spring that they don't get sick with and don't transmit this virus. And yet teachers fight fiercely to keep schools closed, and this reprehensible masking and distancing, and endless cleaning with toxic chemicals for a disease not transmitted by touch.

Fortunately the state doesn't run grocery stores, so they never closed, and there was no outbreak among grocery store clerks.

Why should education be run by the state? When I started writing fiction, I had to think about education, as my background thesis was the need for genius children to get humanity into space. Mathematicians are said to peak in their early 20s, so traditional schools, based on the Prussian model to produce good soldiers, is not ideal. Little kids sit in rows and move to the sounds of bells. Terrible for little boys. If they move around they are labeled as Attention Deficit Disorder and drugged. And the kids at the lower end of the academic spectrum are taught nothing of practical value for the job market. I began to think and write about this in my book series, entitled 'To Slip the Surly Bonds of Earth', now on book four. Initially I was tentative, but watching the unfolding disaster of the last year, clearly state education must be radically rethought.

Q,1. I totally agree. I've been saying for decades the government running schools is the worst education you can get.

A,1. Sadly most people do agree. As soon as they have enough money their kids go to private schools. There is not, after all, anything which the government runs which is run well.

Q,2. So many kids are given terrible advice. They go to university, run up huge debts, and end up with a worthless degree. They seem never to have heard of the Skilled Trades, which guarantees them a good job.

A,2. I tell that to kids all the time. It is difficult to offshore the skilled trades.

Q,3. Elon Musk is right. My cell is my constant companion. It follows my blood O2 as I was anemic and can do an ECG if I want. It asks me if I have fallen if I bang my arm and will call for help if I'm injured. So some of that is good. What is not good is the constant fear mongering by the media. Many seem to be hypnotized by it and believe every word they read. Some people say, 'what's the difference between a chip and your phone, and I don't have a great answer. Where does it end?"

A,3. I have no idea where A.I. will end. If Elon Musk has been sounding the alarm on it for years now. If he is afraid of it, I should be too.

April 8 at 4:58 PM

Here we go again. Another lockdown in Ontario. The Public Health Johnnies (PHJs) and the politicians obviously have never heard of Sweden, which never did lockdown, and Florida which has been open for months. Even the despicable WHO, partly responsible for the disaster, finally advocated against lockdown. As Shakespeare wrote in the play Twelfth Night, 'if it were played upon a stage, I would condemn it as an improbable fiction.'

And one local Ontario PJH has closed schools. Schools have been open for months in Europe. Since spring we have known that kids don't get sick with this virus and they don't transmit. In Canada, as far as I can tell, 1 child under 19, with apparently severe comorbidities, has died of or rather with the virus.

A year of education down the drain; no fun, no sports, no socializing (with these silly masks), no learning about life. No wonder 25% of the kids in the US have contemplated suicide. There is no scientific basis for this, and still they do it. 32 people died in all of Canada yesterday and 19 in Ontario.

Statistics Canada on February 25 indicated no extra deaths in Canada last year. The annual rate of increase actually dropped. In Manitoba there were 9,000 cases: 11,000 had been expected. I also heard that there had been no excess deaths in the US, (hard to believe given all the screams and cries of despair in the media.). To my utter surprise there were no excess deaths in the elderly in Canada. This means that they died with, not of the virus.

90% of all virus deaths in Canada had at least 1 comorbidity (42% being dementia). 100% of deaths under age 45 had comorbidities.

It was surely obvious last summer, when there were virtually no deaths, that this virus was seasonal. A winter resurgence should therefore have been expected. So instead of this summer lockdown and silly masking, excess capacity and cross training medical and nursing staff could have been done. Instead there were no preparations, and in a panic they have just closed my purely elective hospital's operating rooms again, because they anticipate more ICU cases. That lack of planning one sort of expects. But it is the damage done to the kids which is inexplicable.

One wonders how these people can sleep at night, knowing what they are doing to innocent kids. I used to wonder how people would put up with the Red Terror in the Soviet Union, the Holodomor, or Mao's Great Leap Forward, when 30 million people starved to death. But now it is obvious how it happens. People sleep-walk into it. If you want to have nightmares, read Christopher Browning's book 'Ordinary Men', about the atrocities committed in Poland by a Police Battalion, consisting of ordinary men. Those responsible for these futile lockdowns should read Kit Marlowe's 'Faustus' (1590), the man who sold his soul to the Devil.

ADDENDUM

The most important observation ignored by the media and the merchants of doom was the government figures of no excess deaths, even among the elderly, who are at risk from this virus. If there were no excess deaths, then where is this much touted epidemic? This phantom epidemic looks like it is a fevered figment of someone's imagination.

Q,1. I haven't commented on your posts for a bit. I think it is basically because I have given up. I have literally watched my daughter stuck in her bedroom day after day, taking her online courses. She is 25 and trying to finish her degree. What should have been the most exciting last year of school has turned into breathing the same air, day after day. This must end, enough is enough. But how do we stop it? After a whole year of this people are still scared.

Q,2. We are under vicious relentless attack, unable to organize any defense of our country and our freedoms. We stand helpless by, spectators at our own destruction.

A,1. A year ago you might have thought the comments above were from deranged people. But these are sane, sensible women of the world. And I agree with them that the world as we knew it has gone crazy. But what can we do? The people of Germany must have had the same feeling of helplessness in the thirties, or the Soviet Union for almost 70 years, or for that matter Venezuela in the last couple of decades.

April 12 at 5:14 PM

I deeply regret that Shakespeare is no longer taught in what passes for today's state education, either in schools or universities. For how else would you understand the world?

They have just closed schools again in Ontario, Canada. Why? Because 28 people (no data on age or comorbidities), died in all Canada and 15 in Ontario. Still only one sick child under age 19 has died in Canada.

So Macbeth describes the current situation.

'Tomorrow, and tomorrow, and tomorrow
creeps on this petty pace from day to day
Until the end of time.
And all our yesterdays have lighted fools
the way to dusty death.
It is a tale told by an idiot
full of sound and fury, signifying nothing.'

Last spring we were terrified by the propaganda from China, and misinterpretation of statistics by WHO, that the death rate was 3%. But soon we found it 0.3%, bad but survivable. The worldwide relief among the doctors was palpable when in May the Koreans finally showed that if Bat Woman had further weaponized the virus by adding HIV stolen from the Winnipeg lab, it was ineffective. By that time also real scientists, not the global warmists computer modeling types, were educating us all on the Gompertz curve, and it was obvious that the virus was seasonal. They also showed that the Chinese inspired lockdown had no positive effect, was destroying Western economies, and that the collateral deaths from lockdown would far outweighed any possible benefit.

At this stage, the introduction of masking of entire populations in the summer when there were virtually no deaths, indicated that science no longer had anything to do with the response. So I assumed, like most other people, that it was political, in the US to defeat the incumbent, in France to stop the protests against the problems created by the global warmists, and in Canada to let a minority government shovel enormous sums of money out of the door with no parliamentary oversight.

I detailed this in a series of posts, which I noticed were vanishing, along with the information from people I regarded as real experts in the field. Already I could see the true history being turned inside out. So to preserve that record I published them, with many wise and witty comments from my readers, in my book 'Journal of the Plague Year (2020)'. I thought then, with the US election over, that the insanity would disappear.

Sadly, except for Florida, South Dakota, Sweden, and now Texas, I don't see any sign of sanity. Europe is still dancing in and out of lockdown. Like the UK, in the grip of this terrible mutant which has been stalking the land since September 7 people died yesterday; yes! 7 in all the UK.

How can any government or teacher possibly claim that kids and teachers are at risk. They want the vac! Well give it to them, give them all the vac, twice or three times. But they must know that these requirements are unreasonable.

So what's going on? It has been suggested now that it is purely financial. But to do so much harm for money? There is another book worth knowing, which all people in the West used to know, which states, 'what does it profit a man to gain the whole world, but lose his own soul?'

Or was this really WW111, and we lost it, sold out by the elites? All I know is that the posts I am writing now are documenting the inexplicable. I welcome your theories and ideas.

Q,1. I live in Arizona and the governor has declared the state open, but some Democrat cities say they are not. In Phoenix, which has about 4.5 million in the metro area, we have had little or no deaths over the last couple of weeks.

A,1. That is effectively the same in Canada, virtually no deaths and yet the lunatic lockdown continues.

Q,2. The purpose of this Plandemic seems to be to usher in the NWO. How many people has the vaccination killed? No one knows. Is this a way to hurry along depopulation?

Q,3. Some people are actually saying this depopulation business out loud. Not only depopulation, but there is also this crazy plan to dim the sun. I wish that was made up.

A,2. Again, I too wish it was made up. As insane as this sounds, the information the readers are quoting is actually out there, in documented form.

April 17 at 2:26 PM

Where to start? Thinking Yeats
'Things fall apart, The center cannot hold.
The best lack all conviction, while
The worst are full of passionate intensity.
The darkness comes again.
What rough beast, it's hour come at last
slouches towards (Davos? Wuhan?) to be born?

At least some good news. Audio book of book two of my 'To Slip the Surly Bonds of Earth' series, subtitled 'Upon the Further Shore' has just been released. Pretty good. Book one was excellent. Another audio book of mine and Edna Quammie was awful and is being redone. The book is a love story set against the current and future collapse of Europe, with escape to the US and then Mars. What is interesting and sad is to see the collapse occurring as I had imagined.

Also good; just done proofreading a new book, Prions from Wuhan. Written with my friend and scrub nurse, Edna Quammie. We had almost finished before the virus from Wuhan arrived, and quarantine delayed its completion. We chose prions for our bioweapon. If you think that is science fiction, google prions and the Wuhan lab.

Bad news. Hysteria in Canada has reached a new height. This time the sky really is falling, well maybe. Police can stop you on the street. All because of testing. Hard to get figures. One source says 85,000 cases of which 1% are serious. So 99% have no or mild symptoms. Kids don't get sick and don't transmit it. 1 kid with another bad disease has died, so explain to me again just why kids parks are closed.

ICUs are full. Well yes, they are supposed to be. 25% of ICU cases are virus, but with or of? Patients admitted to an ICU can catch the virus there. They are then labeled as a virus case. No one will say what is actually happening. As these figures are based on the PCR test run at 37 to 40x which are completely non diagnostic for illness.

We are being told by the sainted Dr and others that getting the vaccination doesn't let you out of virus jail. Masking, distancing, and lockdown forever. Completely ignoring that lockdown has been shown to be of no value, and wickedly destructive, by 20+ published studies.

Distancing is a joke. 6ft in Canada, 3ft suggested by WHO, fuhgeddaboudit in Florida. And masks. Good news. The post in which I described seeing a lace face mask in the window of a high end ladies lingerie store has been reinstated, as being factual. So I definitely recommend a lace face mask for all, especially little kids. It fulfills the letter of the law, as it is a face covering. Like all other non-filter masks it does no good, but it does a lot less harm than most others. I encourage Victoria's Secret to start production.

The mom and pop stores are closed again, probably for good, and it looks like the schools will return to the failed distance learning. More Pot shops are opening. And you thought Aldous Huxley was making it up when he wrote Brave New World. The Great Reset, the future is here. Sit at home, smoke dope, the government will give you a little food and pocket money, and the media will keep you entertained. That's it. Get used to it. That's the rest of your life. We used to call that house arrest.

For Canadians Florida is a distant dream. Dare I say a beacon of hope!

Q,1. An excellent description of dystopia; although bleak as it is, probably not as hideous as life will become if the Great Reset juggernaut rolls on unimpeded.

Q,2. I don't know how or why the populace has become so fearful, so set on hiding from this virus. The media I suppose is likely the culprit. What is new is that we now live with this constant source of information in our hands and our pockets. It is inescapable, this constant barrage of fearful non-information. Non, because most of it is based on speculation, misinformation, because of the need to get those clicks. The young are most at risk here as they have been raised with this media and follow it as gospel. What a sad world!

A,2. I think that this is a good explanation. Never before have we had immediate news constantly at our fingertips. That also might explain why the young believe this nonsense so fervently. The people in my clinic who believe it least, seem to be those from Eastern Europe who lived under communism and know all about the constant barrage of false information promulgated by the government.

April 21 at 5:05 PM

Another good man down! Tony Hedley, an old friend, and well known hip surgeon has just passed on. There is sorrow, but death is part of life. It is not really how we die; it is more how we lived. Kipling wrote,

'for each man hears as the twilight nears
to the beat of his dying heart,
the Devil drum on the window pane,
you did it, but was it art?'

For Tony it was art, a life well lived. I met him in the 80s when modern joint replacement was in its infancy. My engineering buddy, Bob Pilliar and I had developed the technology to anchor metal implants to bone in the 70s. It takes years and hundreds of experiments to get from the laboratory into widespread clinical use, which makes people understandably a little nervous about the current vaccine.

In the 80s modern joint replacement was so new the world had to be taught how to do it. A relatively small group of surgeons, mostly American, had to go and teach it. We called ourselves the Traveling Road Show. You can read about our adventures, thrills and spills, the laughter, and the tears, and how that changed medical education, in my book. Google the title, 'Have Knife Will Travel.' Because that is what we did. I was in the air, flying somewhere once every 2 or 3 weeks for 30+ years, lecturing and demonstrating surgery.

Modern joint replacement surgery is expensive, so initially only a few countries could afford it, like the US, Europe, Japan, and South Korea. We were consultants for the half a dozen major implant companies. We used to bump into each other in places like the Shilla hotel in Seoul or the airport lounge in Narita, Tokyo.

Tony ran a major conference in Phoenix annually for years. He would complain that it took a week for his headache to go away after we left, after many late nights of laughter, drinking, boasting, and lying.

Those were the days when travel was fun. It all ended with the fall of the twin towers. The terrorists wanted to damage the West, and they succeeded, permanently it seems. We shuffle shoeless through airports 20 years after one incompetent shoe bomber.

Travel is now miserable, except on a cruise ship, as long as you don't bother getting off where it docks.

Thinking of cruise boats, it is so sad that the Public Health Johnnies (PHJs) have ignored the data from the Diamond Princess, which was a perfect experiment, where so few died of the virus, all elderly. The PHJs ignored the evidence in front of their eyes and brought in lockdown, the worst public health disaster in all history. By doing their best to prevent spread during the safe summer, when Vitamin D levels were high and UV light reduced the dose of virus, they encouraged the second wave by limiting population immunity.

Oh well, summer is almost here, but sadly in Toronto it is snowing. I so wish the global warmists were correct. Imagine Toronto 3 or 4 degrees warmer. 'Bliss would it be

- -'.

Q,1. It is not a public health crisis, it is a public policy crisis. If they had done nothing, the outcome would not have been worse, and our economy wouldn't be in shambles.

Q,2. If they had done nothing, essentially like Sweden, the outcomes would have been far better in terms of loss of life years.

A,1@2. The data on the virus survival from Sweden is certainly much better than Canada or the US.

Q,3. It looks like a long summer ahead. I feel so sorry for the young people whose lives are normally full of socializing, parties, and laughter in the warm months. They are missing so much.

A.3. The young are being crucified for a disease which has hardly touched them. For the young, a single summer is a lifetime.

Q,4. Condolences for you friend. He will be pleased that he lives on in your fond memories. And thanks for my new knee.

April 24 at 12:38 PM

Lockdown again! Government virus snoopers are all over. One came to the medical clinic threatening us. 'We see too many patients.' Since March last year, all patients have been screened by a doctor before admission. Any virus symptoms or contacts refused entry until clear. I wrote then that the clinic manager was doing a better job than the utterly incompetent feds who were still allowing flights in from China. There have been no virus cases traced to this clinic, not a single one.

So now, because of this bumptious health Jenny, my elderly arthritic patients have to limp almost a city block to another building, back for X-rays, then back again. And this is science, when the big box stores are full?

It was this time last year when I found freedom had gone. I had a post that disappeared because I named the heroine Ai Fen. Interesting to see if this is still a trigger. I was shocked, but I should have known. I had been watching freedoms slowly disappearing for decades. I wrote about its loss with Edna Quammie, my long term scrub nurse and friend, in our book 'The Big House, Toronto General Hospital from 1972 to 1984.' We watched it happen, but never found a hill to die on. When you wake up, it is too late, it is all gone. As Kipling wrote, 'gone, gone, gone with lost Atlantis.'

The Enlightenment, that peculiar Western concept which arose nowhere else, that an individual was an individual with intrinsic worth, and not part of a herd, a hive, or a collective, burst into being in the 1700s. It lasted 300 glorious years but has faded away. As Thomas Jefferson wrote, 'democracy is great, if you can keep it.'

But democracy depends on free speech and that is long gone. No person in Canada or most of the West who works in education, the Arts, government, or most large companies has any right to free speech.

And these new clinic rules, we can't even complain. No one in authority has read the 20+ publications showing lockdown is of no value and is the biggest Public Health disaster in living memory. These incompetents Public Health Johnnies have never heard of Sweden or Florida.

I realized last summer that this had nothing to do with science, when lockdown continued, interfering with a safe summer spread, when high vitamin D improved immunity and UV light reduced virus load. Continued lockdown encouraged mutations, reduced natural vitamin D from sunshine and therefore worsened exposure of the ill elderly.

When I arrived in Toronto in the early 70s it was bursting with life; the young immigrants had escaped the dead hands of socialism. It was wildly exciting, blue sky thinking, make money, make love, work like crazy, eat the world alive. I wrote about that joyous time in my book 'Have Knife Will Travel.' The kids of today have no idea about the wild times their grandparents had. Then it all seeped away, as the administrative class of has-beens and never-wasses took over.

Where will it end? The voices of reason and science have been silenced, one after another. If the myth of global warming survived Climategate, when the untruths were shown to all, then what hope is left?

Oh well, we have been there before. Last time we called it the Dark Ages. What will we call it this time?

Q,1. Add doctors to that list of people denied free speech. I was told by a friend, a GP, that the virus dies quickly on hard surfaces, so all this repeated cleaning is worthless. Then he said, 'don't tell anyone I said that.' I was stunned. He told me that once you have recovered from this virus you can't get it again and can't spread it. He told me that if people knew he was saying these things he could lose his career.

A,1. He is correct. Look at the young doctor in New York who pointed out that ventilators were killing people, who only needed positive pressure oxygen, like a CPAP machine for sleep apnea. He was fired. Many other docs have been fired for talking out about the value of the drugs which cannot be named. And your doc is absolutely right about all this ridiculous cleaning with toxic chemicals. This virus is not spread by contact.

April 28 at 12:19 PM

Terrible day. 2 gas stations from 2 companies managed to screw up 2 credit cards. Then a Ministry of Health Johnny snooping about the medical clinic disturbing patients and creating chaos.

Thinking of Fermat's last theorem. Are bureaucrats born awful or does becoming a bureaucrat make them awful? Contact with these people brings to mind Hannah Arendt's book The Banality of Evil, about Adolph Eichmann, the banal little bureaucrat who failed at everything except genocide.

Lockdown is arguably the greatest Public Health disaster in all Western history. What fueled it? I examined these issues very cautiously, afraid of being canceled, in my book Journal of the Plague Year(2020). The reason for the escape / release/ spread of the virus is obvious. The response in some countries was clearly political/ financial/ and backed by some public service unions. But that doesn't wholly explain the ferocity of the bureaucrat. We were all fooled initially by the propaganda videos from Wuhan of people dropping dead in the street, but soon realized that was all fake. So did the bureaucrats in the CDC actually continue to believe this, or did they and WHO have other motives?

One US state has mandatory masking of kids 2 years and up. Even WHO says kids 5 and over. Don't they know that kids don't get sick with this virus and they don't transmit? Sweden never did masking and they have done better than most countries.

Good news. I went to 2 separate banks to sort out the credit cards. The girl tellers were so sweet, so helpful and so efficient. Just when you think that the world is full of thieves and jackasses, your faith is restored, by banks of all places!

More good news. As a surgeon I have worn a mask for 50+ years. Ask any OR nurse who has also used them for years. A wet, soiled, reused mask spreads infection. The bureaucrats mandating masking, like the sainted Dr, clearly have no idea. Finland has just decided no mandatory masking. Better than nothing, but they could have asked Sweden a year ago. Even the utterly incompetent CDC says no masking outdoors after the vaccine. But how about none at all, especially after the vac?

Other good news. The Indian outbreak is a Casedemic as they have ramped up testing of asymptomatic people using the PCR test at a 40x multiplier. That should produce a billion positive tests. The much touted Oxygen shortage there is chronic, not new.

Thinking about last year, was the lockdown with economic destruction of the West phase 1 of WW111, and we lost, without realizing it? The Greens are now back in full force planning to destroy what is left of the world's economy, outside China. Are they phase 11 of this war?

Q, You surmise correctly dear Author. The awakening is occurring though. Let's hope it does not pan out to be too little, too late

A, I wish, but I fear, "low among the alders lie the derelict foundations' of the West. Or as T.S. Elliot wrote,

'Eyes, there are no eyes here
In this valley of dying stars,
This hollow valley,
this broken jaw of our lost kingdom.
This is the way the world ends,
Not with a bang, but a whimper.'

May 1

Guess what? I have just learned that the CT (cycle threshold) used for the PCR test in Ontario is 42. What this means is that a tiny fragment of protein, hopefully but not necessarily, from a Coronavirus, is multiplied until it can be identified. A CT of 20, which is used in Singapore, means multiplied about a billion times, so there probably is some living virus present. It doesn't mean that you are sick or even know you have it. A CT of 42 means it is amplified about a trillion times, yes, a trillion. So has no real diagnostic significance.

Add the likelihood of some lab contamination. Also remember that there is a 1% false positive. What this means is that if the positive rate is 2%, half the positive tests were negative. A new industry has developed with the huge number of these expensive tests being done worldwide. So there is a huge perverse incentive for someone to over-test and over-diagnose.

I hesitate to comment on ICUs other than to point out that they are so expensive they are always almost full. They can usually function at 20% overcapacity, so having 10% capacity left, actually means 30%.

And virus deaths, with or of? Again in some countries there is a huge incentive for the death certificate to read died of the virus, not with it. In the US it is a financial incentive. If you test positive and a month later die of a heart attack, guess what your death certificate will likely say? Look at the excess mortality from year to year. And remember if it was low one year there's lots of 'dry tinder' as it is called, for next year. For some countries last year there was no excess above the norm. So in reality, the virus had essentially no effect. Some Pandemic eh?

I hesitate to write about the development of mutants for fear of the dreaded algorithm. But consider how to do 'gain of function' in the lab. If this is ignored, I may speculate tentatively on how lockdown has stimulated this.

And masking! The sainted Dr wears 2 after the vaccine. The theater of the absurd. A wet mask will aerosolize the particles, making more, not less. Masking little kids is inhuman. A wet, dirty piece of cloth on a little kid's face all day, so they can't learn how to read facial expressions. Why? The virus doesn't affect kids and they don't transmit. Or at least this version doesn't. If lockdown continues, watch this space.

I thought that this would end with the US election, but now other factors are at play. So I am collecting for my next book, Journal of the Pseudo-Plague Year(2021). I used many of your funny and acerbic comments in the first book. So I would appreciate more comments for the next one.

Q,1. Guess we ought to follow the money. There are fortunes being made in PPE, tests and all the other paraphernalia to be used by business and industry. I would really like to know the connections, if any, of elected officials to businesses raking in the dough.

A,1. One is awfully well connected to a certain leading official in Ottawa. I know of another. If I know this, and I take no interest in what is happening in Ottawa, then many others must know also. But sadly, nothing is being said by the legacy media.

Q,2. The PCR test was never meant to be used as a diagnostic tool. It is way too sensitive for that. I am not saying the virus doesn't exist, but with a survival rate of in excess of 99% it can hardly be called a deadly killer.

A,2. The man who got the Nobel prize for developing it, always said that it must not be used in this way. He also said that, used with a CT of 40 you can find anything. He had numerous quarrels with the sainted Dr, who he said, knew very little about anything. If interested, just google his name. The videos are very edifying.

May 5

Is the tide turning? More excellent docs appearing on social media. Look at them quickly as they may not last long. I dare not mention names for fear of censorship. They compare our response to this virus to the Salem Witch trials or the Children's Crusade. A video has just surfaced of the same fear mongers trying to stir up the same hysteria about H1N1 years ago. But no one believed them then, so nothing happened, and the H1N1 vaccine disappeared. This time the legacy media and big tech helped them.

Fear porn is everywhere, for an invisible disease, which in most cases, you only know you have if a totally unreliable test says you have it. If a PCR test run at 40x says you have something, then your family and contacts must have the same unreliable, expensive test. Ponzi would be proud.

Children are super-spreaders; except they are not. 4 kids under 19 in Canada have died, one with leukemia and one for lack of medical care. They have not released information on the other two.

Teachers are at risk; except they are not. There is as yet no documented case of a student infecting a teacher. Junior schools never closed in Sweden and have been open in Europe for months.

Bars and restaurants will kill you, except in Florida.

Unbelievably, the Precautionary Principle has taken over our lives. Briefly it means 'take action without knowing what action to take.' Or 'jump down from the fence and ride madly off in all directions.' Taken logically, ban cars. For healthy people under 50 a car is far more dangerous than the virus.

Follow 'the' science, they bleat. But who's science? Social distancing in Canada 6ft, WHO 3ft, Florida fuhgeddaboudit. And masks? The only evidence is that universal masking is not of any benefit, and on kids is worse than useless.

Traditional Western medicine has been ignored. If you are sick, stay at home. Making everyone stay at home is silly as that is where most virus spread occurs. Universal lockdown, if it does anything, increases the risk to the vulnerable and encourages mutants.

In northern countries most people are low in vit D. I used to take 1,000 iu. but now believe 4,000 iu in the winter. Strangely the Canadian minister of Health disagrees!! Other well-known supplements and drugs, often OTC in other countries, cannot even be mentioned by name. In Ontario docs have been warned of disciplinary action if we say anything contrary to official policy. The Canadian feds are trying to pass a new bill to censor all social media communications such as this post. How sad. This used to be a free country.

Whatever purpose lockdown originally had has long since disappeared. Many publications have shown no value. The deaths due to lockdown have yet to be tabulated because a missed cancer diagnosis won't show up this year. Eventually collateral deaths will far outweigh those from the virus

Q,1. Ponzi would be proud. Yes, I think so too. Docs, pharmacists, and even first responders are afraid of losing their careers if they question anything. I went to see my doc two weeks ago for a blood test. He said it is difficult right now and he will do the test in six months.

Q,2. It is getting a little better. Six months ago the face mask guards outside a store took their job seriously. Now they shrug their shoulders, apologize, and commiserate as they know it is silly.

Q,3. I saw a video where they were trying to do exactly the same thing in the 70s with swine flu.

A,1. I know they tried to do the same thing with H1N1 in 2009. But Der Spiegel, the German newspaper, pointed out that there were thousands of positive tests but no sick people, so the scam collapsed. Curiously, the same people who are involved today were involved then. What I found out later was that that vaccine was producing narcolepsy which was one of the reasons it was pulled off the market. I took that vaccine as I believed the epidemic was serious. But I had no knowledge of any side effects until now.

May 10

Listening to a senior Swedish doc being grilled by a hostile interviewer. Using whatever metric you like, Sweden, with no lockdown, did pretty well during the pandemic. Lord Beaconsfield said that there are lies, damned lies, and statistics. This interviewer had them all. He even tried to claim that the ludicrous modeling done by the Imperial College, which terrified the gullible Public Health Johnnies (PHJs), was correct. They were even less realistic than the models of the Global Warmists, who sadly are again raising their wickedly destructive voices.

I would like to say that I don't understand people like that interviewer, but sadly I do, we all do. The legacy media breeds them. This is how they come out of journalism school, as products of the Long March of the Frankfurt School. By this time they surely know that the PCR test run at 42CT, has only a passing relationship to reality, about an invisible disease you don't know you have unless the test tells you.

So what's the motivation behind this charade of closing mom and pop stores, unless they are selling pot, and why the masking of children? Does anyone take seriously our chief PHJ who says you must wear a mask during sex? The masked jogger that one frequently sees running down an empty street absolutely does!

A major Australian news outlet is drawing attention to documents which actually have been available for a year or more regarding the origin and purpose of the virus. And yet no one has asked the sainted Dr just why he took it on himself to fund this 'gain of function' research in a military lab in a potentially hostile country.

Forget this PCR test fantasy and look at the deaths, recognizing that a death within 28 days of a positive test is counted as a virus death, which means vast exaggeration. As we enter summer in the North, death rates are dropping. In the UK 2 died yesterday and yet lockdown continues. Has this really anything to do with the virus? In Canada 39 died yesterday, 2 in Alberta. And yet we have the shameful sight of an Alberta pastor on his knees on a highway being shackled and dragged away.

So will this change society forever? We find that the sturdy and independent yeomanry are neither, and will carry out orders, no matter how obscene. I had always planned to read Christopher Browning's book 'Ordinary Men' about the atrocities committed by a regular German police battalion in Poland during the Holocaust. But now I don't need to. You can see it happening in front of your own eyes. A pastor dragged off in chains, another Dietrich Bonhoeffer. In Canada!

On the 10th of Nov 1917, 17,000 young Canadians were killed or wounded in the battle of Passchendaele, for what? To preserve a government which drags men of God off in chains? What would these heroes think of this travesty?

John McCrae wrote about the poppies in Flanders fields, and the torch of freedom,

'To you we fling the torch
Be yours to hold it high.'

I don't think a pastor in chains is holding the torch high.

Q,1. I saw the unnecessary humiliation and roughness with the pastor, and the disruption of all the traffic on the road. I wonder if the police were told to behave in that barbaric fashion, or did they just figure it out on their own!

Q,2. Our church is only allowed ten people to attend each service. And yet as many as you like in a big box store, and no limits on numbers at a good riot. And this has something to do with science?

Q,3. Here in Southern California our church has finally opened back up with no mask requirement. One has to wonder what role the attempted recall of this despicable governor has played in reducing his version of "The Science."

A,1. It is difficult to understand this desperate desire to close churches. Perhaps the use of a 'common cup,' be halted during a pandemic, but why anything else. Perhaps it is an attempt to prevent people contemplating with others the lunacy of what is currently happening.

May 14

Shakespeare nailed it again as Hamlet described the response to the virus:

'the whips and scorns of time,
The rich man's contumely,
the oppressor's wrong,
the insolence of office.'

Maybe add the utter incompetence of office.

In Toronto the Taste of the Danforth, a glorious annual summer street festival of Greek food, drink, music and dance, Gay Pride Parade, and the wonderful colorful festival of Caribbean culture have just been cancelled by the politicians and Public Health Johnnies (PHJs).

They fail to understand or care about the summer sunshine increase in vitamin D levels, enhancing immunity, and the UV light reducing the virus load. Go riot all you want, but have some clean, safe, legal fun - No Way! Fun and happiness after a long winter in Canada, the coldest country on earth-. Nein! Absolutely verboten in this era of Fear Porn. If people were happy they might stop listening to the muddled merchants of despair, the PHJs.

The only philosophers I ever thought knew what they were talking about were Hobbes and Hume. The last year, especially for children, as described by Hobbes was 'nasty, brutish and short.' Their youth has been ruined by uncaring bureaucrats and legacy media. David Hume pointed out how 'easy it is for the few to manipulate the many,' especially with fear porn. The legacy media and others followed Joseph Goebbels philosophy, 'repeat the lie often enough and people will believe it.'

But just maybe Kant was right, that 'truth will out.' The actual origins of the virus and the funding of it is slowly being talked about. We have known about it for a long time and I wrote about it very circumspectly, in my book Journal of the Plague Year(2020). The sainted Dr is being asked for the first time why the legal ban on 'gain of function', that extremely dangerous activity, was ignored, and why it was moved offshore to a country potentially no friend of the West.

What is even worse was the French, who designed the lab in Wuhan, withdrew as the local contractors were not following international specs. It is rumored that rather than the level 4, some of the work was done in a level 2 facility, about as secure as a dentist's office. Early videos showed leaking storage fridges and totally unprotected staff at work.

Another tragedy was that the politicians and the legacy media believed the propaganda from China, aided by WHO and the CDC, that the hitherto inconceivable lockdown cured the virus in 2 weeks. So we 'flattened the curve', and a year later in Canada, are still flattening the curve.

All the evidence that lockdown was the greatest public health disaster in history continues to be ignored. Doubtless it will continue over the summer by ramping up the PCR multiplier, until there is a fall resurgence in what is now an endemic virus.

Q,1. Caribana is canceled for the second year. The huge crowds at events in Florida indicates how unnecessary this cancellation was

Q,2. The theater of the absurd. It is hard to beat the bard. He described it all.

A,1@2. The lunacy continues, closed schools, churches, lockdown, and masking. Makes you think of the song,

'When will they ever learn?' or perhaps rephrase, 'when will they ever care?'

May 20

Just released, new book, available on Amazon, etc. the title is 'Prions from Wuhan'. Prions make a virus look like a nice guy. Google Mad Cow Disease if you want nightmares.

For no obvious reason, in the face of a virus which was tightly targeted at the ill elderly only (average age of virus deaths in Sweden was over 80, most with comorbidities, especially dementia), the West, influenced by WHO and the CDC, threw out all we knew of medicine and followed communist China's propaganda about lockdown.

We know who funded the 'gain of function' research in Wuhan, which turned a harmless bat virus into a killer, and we know who is funding the Anthrax research. But who is funding the prion research in Wuhan? These things are not living so cannot be killed except at high temperatures. There are no tests, no treatment, and you don't know you have the disease for a couple of years, and then it takes another 2 years or so to die. Hopefully it will never be released.

Turning to our old friend coronavirus, the 2 weeks to flatten the curve is now over a year. Toronto is trying for the world lockdown record. Canada already has one record. Our chief Public Health Jenny insists that a mask be worn during sex. Sadly she was not joking. Listening to another august PHJ prognosticating a resurgence if schools open. Sadly our Canadian PHJs seem unaware that schools in Europe and Florida have been open with no increase. And they still mask kids, in spite of knowing for a year that kids don't get sick with this one and they don't transmit. And when will they ever look at the data which shows no positive effect of lockdown? Instead, it is the biggest Public Health disaster in history. The long term effects of missed cancer diagnosis, deferred surgeries, education loss, emotional damage, and economic loss have yet to play out.

Karl Popper pointed out that one negative fact destroys a nice theory, and Sweden and Florida destroyed the theory of lockdown and masking. Now that the global Warmists are starting to bellow again, about the Great Reset, another one of Popper's sayings is worth thinking about. He said, 'those who promise paradise on earth never produced anything but hell.'

I so hope that I am wrong but 'build back better,' with it's expensive unpredictable energy, seems to me like a step back into the Dark ages, with poverty, hunger, violence, and despair.

Q,1. Flawed humans should not push their agendas on others. Previous attempts at Utopia have always ended in disaster.

A,1. I could not put it better myself. The killing fields of Cambodia or the gulags of the Soviets. As Thomas Gray wrote,

'To wade through slaughter to a throne
And close the gates of mercy on mankind.'

May 24

Listening to J (names carry the risk of deletion). He said that Canada, like New Zealand, has decided on zero virus, complete eradication. I had no idea. No PHJ ever said so, but for the last year Jay has been correct, so maybe. But the idea of complete eradication of the virus is simply silly.

Two viruses have been eradicated, rinderpest in cattle and Smallpox in humans. But Smallpox had no animal reservoir; it was a purely human disease. It was readily recognizable, with the pox, which left horrible scars and was very lethal. The last case was in Bangladesh in the 70s I think. Authorities still keep the vaccine in case a rogue nation releases it again as a bioweapon.

The virus from Wuhan was tightly targeted at the ill elderly. For most healthy people it is not serious, and often you need a test to know you have had it. It is highly infectious in an indoor setting such as lockdown and is airborne, so masks and distancing have little or no effect. So how can it possibly be eliminated?

Even if the vaccine is forced on every man, woman and baby, there is still an animal reservoir, cats, and dogs and even a tiger in the Bronx zoo, and if the sainted Dr is to be believed, even in poor bats living 1,000k from Wuhan. So are you going to vac them all? I mean, give your head a shake!

I am not anti vac. For 30+ years I was flying internationally once every 2 or 3 weeks teaching modern hip and knee replacement surgery. I told that tale of triumphs and disasters in my book 'Have Knife Will Travel.' I got every vaccine known to man. The only ones that made me sick were cholera or typhoid, I forget which. Those had short immunity and had to be repeated. Hygiene is now good enough in most countries, so these are not necessary. All my kids got all their vaccines. But this one? I don't know. Especially for kids who are at no risk of dying of the virus

To eliminate the virus, you will also need an effective test and trace. This is possible with a lethal disease, spread by contact only, like Ebola, or a permanently sealed island like New Zealand, as long as it is kept sealed. It is not possible with a highly infectious, low mortality, airborne disease, already present worldwide.

And quarantine! This was developed in Venice to keep out the plague. The infected sailing ships had to remain at an island in the lagoon for 40 days, hence the name. For a highly infectious, low morbidity disease already widespread in a country, it makes no sense.

And this fear about double or triple mutants! Viruses mutate to become more infectious and less lethal.

Thankfully it is now becoming possible to listen to people who know what they are talking about. And the sainted Dr and his merry band at the CDC are being asked just why they provided funds to a certain lab in Wuhan, where it turns out the actual work was being done in a level 2 lab, which is about as secure as a dentist's office. What is worrying is that there are moves afoot to fund more 'gain of function', presumably in the same leaky lab.

May 29

Is there no hope for the widow's son? I was lecturing in Braunschweig, a few klicks from the border in November of 1989. At midnight news came that the wall was down. I remember the sense of relief that the long nightmare of Socialism was over, and the West was spared.

I had the same feeling of hope when news came that social media would no longer censor any mention of the virus origin.

What most people don't know is that what terrified many docs was that we knew that several Chinese scientists were deported from Canada in the fall of 2019, and we in Canada don't deport even murderers. Among other things, the HIV virus had been stolen from the level 4 lab in Winnipeg and sent to Wuhan. The great fear was that Bat Woman had added HIV to the horseshoe bat virus in addition to the ability to infect humans, which she was known to have added years before. If so, there would be no immunity ever.

Initial studies from Korea suggested that was the case in 20%. It was only in late May of 2020 that they showed these were late excreters and had immunity. The worldwide relief was palpable.

It was obvious that the virus was tightly targeted at the ill elderly and those with comorbidities. Children and the productive were spared. Almost as if it were tailored to reduce the number of pensioners who are a major problem in China as a result of the one child policy.

There never was any scientific basis for lockdown, and it has repeatedly been shown to be utterly useless. The collateral damage is immense, with millions at risk of food insecurity, missed medical treatments, poverty, marital discord, child abuse, and despair. And yet inexplicably it continues in some places, notably Canada.

And mandatory masking last summer, when people were outside in the sunshine and when immunity is at its highest in the north. It made no sense then. Maybe it was to prolong the fear until the fall and winter resurgence of a seasonal virus. We thought the examples of Florida and Texas would get rid of this useless masking.

But today I have just seen that Health Canada has a new mandate to continue masking, indoors and outdoors, even after the vaccine. Even the CDC has finally admitted that masking after the vaccine is not necessary. The sainted Dr continues a strenuous rearguard action, but he seems a little distracted trying to distance himself from his funding of 'gain of function research' in what turned out to be a level 2 lab in Wuhan, which is about the safety level of a nails salon.

So in Canada everyone, including the poor innocent kids, will continue to be masked, faceless, frightened, and uneducated. This from a country whose young men stormed Vimy Ridge and in the thousands gave their lives for freedom. Looking down from above, they must wonder why they bothered.

So what's the end game here? You tell me.

Q,1. A note from California. Went to Arizona last week for a much needed reminder of what freedom looks and feels like. The simple things were wonderful, walking around with no masks, talking to people, going into restaurants. Come on Canada, you too can take your masks off.

A,1. I wish, but contrary to all logic, they have just reinforced the mask mandate, even after getting the vaccine. This clearly has no longer has anything to do with the virus. I just so wish I had kept my Florida medical license.

Q,2. I don't see this ending well. Once authoritarian types get control, it's pretty much over.

A.2. Sadly that is true. 200 Bolsheviks took over Russia in 1917 and held all Eastern Europe in prison for seventy years. Castro inc. still rules Cuba, and the CCP China.

June 3

Hardly surprising, schools in Ontario are to remain closed, with no guarantee that they will open in the fall. There may after all, be new variants, double, triple, or tooth fairy. As expected, these lockdowns expedited the development of variants, which are likely more infectious but certainly no more lethal. Oh, and by the way, once 300 or so kids have been trialed, all kids will be given the vaccine. Tragically over a year lost from school, and now this.

Thinking of Wilfred Owen in despair in WW1, the youth being sacrificed for what? So a whole country could be in lockdown for over a year?

'Strange friend,' said I, 'here is no cause to mourn.'

'None,' said the other. 'None save the undone year,

the hopelessness.'

Listening on the car radio on the way to work, this political prattle of following 'the' science. As soon as you qualify something, you change it. 'The Science' ceased to be science when governments ignored the scandal of Climategate and carried merrily on to ban cheap reliable energy. Somehow the belief that CO2 is a poison, not a plant food, continues.

Fortunately 'the' science of the pandemic is starting to fall apart. The wheels are coming off the sainted Dr and his many tales. Even the credulous legacy media is beginning to wonder why the sainted Dr funded incredibly dangerous 'gain of function' research in a country who is not our friend. And in what turned out to be not the level 4 lab, but a level 2, which has about the same security as the meat counter in a food store. The theory of the heroic bat which flew 1,000k to end up in someone's soup, does now seem a little unlikely.

Listening to some clever US/ German lawyers who have begun a class action lawsuit on behalf of the bankrupt mom and pop stores. Sadly, the first case in Canada was dismissed, but is under appeal. There have been some successes in Europe. The main challenge is the use of the PCR test. The Nobel prize winner, the man who developed this test, said it was never to be used for diagnosis of illness. But with a little Berlin twist, based supposedly on a genome sent from China, and a very big CT, and some boosting from the ever honest WHO, all countries began to use it.

As most people now know, a small fragment of protein, possibly from a coronavirus, of which at least four produce one form of the common cold, is multiplied. In Singapore 20x is accepted, but in Canada we use 42x, roughly a trillion magnifier. Many scientists say that 90% of positive tests with that multiplier means no symptoms. When I was a medical student a long time ago, if you had no symptoms and you were not sick, you didn't have the disease.

We have known this for over a year and yet the charade continues. All patients admitted to hospital are tested and retested. If they test positive they are labeled as a COVID case, even if the original problem was a broken leg. Deaths are similar. Did they die with it or of it, or was it the ventilator that killed them?

News leaking out of Israel about the vaccine. I can't say more as docs in Ontario will lose their license if they don't spout the party line. And the Canadian/ US border is still closed. No one knows why. Unless you fly either way or drive in from the US. And somehow someone is pretending this is science?

Ah well, just keep the fear going for another few months, and the Fall resurgence, and the Ottawa tooth fairy variant will allow ongoing lockdown. And you thought 1984 and the Brave New World were fiction. If you want to read another likely scenario, google my book series 'To Slip the Surly Bonds of Earth.'

Q,1. What is going on with these vaccines? I hear all sorts of problems. They stop one being used then start again. One must be used in this age group and not another. Every day it is something different.

A,1. What is so disturbing is that doctors in Ontario have been threatened by their licensing body that if we say anything about the vaccines we may lose our license to practice medicine. It begs the question of what is the problem which must be covered up? We know that the adverse effects of the vaccine are almost impossible to report, so no one has any idea.

Q,2. When will these so-called variants be named correctly? The Propaganda variant, Tyranny variant, Hypocrisy variant, Liar variable, Communist variant.

Q,3. Joseph Goebbels would be proud.

Q,4. So true and so sad. So many have drunk the Kool-Aid. These vaccines are still experimental.

A,2. And this PCR test can distinguish between the variants? I don't think so. I have heard it can't distinguish between a variant and a common cold variant, alive or dead.

June 7

Kit Marlowe wrote in Tamburlaine,

'Is it not passing brave to be a king

and ride in triumph through Persepolis.'

Every kid should have his Kit Marlowe moment. Mine was almost 60 years ago when I won the British Junior Hammer Throw.

The tragedy is that currently universities in the Anglo-sphere are so ideologically driven and degenerate, that I recommend kids go to a trade school. I believe it is possible to graduate in the humanities without reading Shakespeare or Kit Marlowe. He died in 1593 at age 29. Imagine the possibilities if he had lived.

If you know Marlowe's work 'The Tragic History of Dr Faustus,' you might have some understanding of what is happening today. In eerily similar circumstances Faustus, even the names are similar, sold his soul to Mephistopheles (the devil), for forbidden knowledge.

Over the last few years someone sold out to the devil for 'gain of function' to make a harmless bat virus into a killer. Who knows what will come next from these leaking fridges in that level 2 lab in Wuhan. My coauthor Edna Quammie and I speculated in our new book 'Prions From Wuhan.'

It looks as if the wheels are coming off the coverup, just as they did with Dr Faustus, when the devil came to take him to Hell.

'Now thou hast but one bare hour to live

the clock will strike.

The devil will come

and Faustus must be damn'd.'

It is only just now possible to talk openly about the origin of the virus. But how safe is it to tell the other truths? I mean it was no great secret where it came from. The mystery was the utterly inexplicable reaction of most of the world. People ask, 'why didn't docs speak up?' Well, think how many brave docs lost their jobs and reputation, and in China probably paid the ultimate price. For a while I felt alone, a simple orthopedic surgeon with an obsolete iPhone trying to work out what was going on. As some of my posts were being disappeared I published them in book form 'Journal of the Plague Year(2020). Just google the title. If I had a young family and a mortgage I would probably have kept my mouth shut also. In Ontario, Canada, docs are being threatened with loss of medical license if they say anything contrary to the official guidelines which are those of the CCP and WHO.

But it is starting to look better. Everywhere now I look on the net I find brilliant, knowledgeable docs and scientists beginning to make plain what is happening. Quite frankly, it is very, very concerning.

I was always taught to assume stupidity before malevolence, but stupidity only takes you so far. We have known since last spring that the virus was tightly targeted at the ill elderly. Kids and the healthy young were never at risk. The sickness rate of unprotected grocery store clerks was close to zero. And still lockdown continued, knowing that it had absolutely no effect on virus transmission, except possibly encouraging it, as most transmission was at close quarters indoors. It was a Public Health disaster. We will be paying the price for this lunacy for years with deaths from despair, cancer and others in developed countries, and starvation, HIV, TB, and malaria in lesser developed.

Why were simple, safe, cheap, and relatively effective medications banned? Why did the Canadian federal minister of Health recently state that Vit D had no role? Eh? Ignorance or orders?

So the mystery is not the virus, it is the wholly inexplicable reaction to it. The sums of money are so vast that the truth may be hard to come by.

Q,1. One reader sent a photo of the four horsemen of the apocalypse labeled with the names of the four big pharmas.

A,1. I cannot reproduce it here, but it is certainly worth a look. Big pharma and public health have completely lost any credibility they ever had. And I say that as one who until this recent fiasco believed in them and defended them.

June 12

Out walking. 25*C and bright sunshine. Park empty except for a mother and child, both masked. Adults can do what they want. That is no concern of mine. But a poor little 3 or 4 year old child wearing a wet soiled mask. This is child abuse. And yet, how can you blame the mother with the relentless pressure from the legacy media to wear a mask at all times.

Just looking at the political leaders meeting on a beach in England, in the open air, in the sunshine. All of them claim to have been vaccinated. And yet our dear leader of Canada is wearing a virtue signaling face mask. So how can you blame the poor child's mother?

And to watch this bunch of doofuses doing elbow bumps. God help us all. I guess that the charade is not about to end soon.

Everyone who wears a mask for a living, like a surgeon, an operating room nurse, or drywaller knows a little about them. Unlike Public Health Johnnies (PHJ), who clearly know nothing. A paint sprayer uses a filter mask, as do docs dealing with a respiratory infection. They fit tightly and are uncomfortable. A surgeon uses a mask so he doesn't drool into the wound. If it gets wet or soiled it is changed immediately and is not reused.

The emails recently released show that even the sainted Dr F knew that mandatory masking was useless, and yet he kept pushing it. Even after he claimed he was vaccinated himself. Why? And if one mask was useless then use 2 or 3. All a great charade. What more foolishness can you get the public to swallow?

The tragedy is that thousands knew that mandatory masking, brought in in the middle of last summer, was just silly. Or worse, led to more infection, as did lockdown. Maybe the PHJs did not know. I find it increasingly difficult to discover what they do know. It doesn't seem like much. But any voices of dissent were silenced.

The emails also show collaboration between the sainted Dr and the so-called social media fact checkers. A classic case one would have thought of the fox guarding the henhouse.

We are now able to state without fear of being canceled, the origin of the virus. We also know that the sainted Dr was funding, via a circuitous route, this 'gain of function' research to make a harmless bat virus deadly for a tightly targeted group of humans. This research had been banned in the US, so the sainted Dr moved it offshore by funding it in a country not exactly the best friend of the West. Was this naivety or a Benedict Arnold moment? As they don't teach history, at least in Canada, the ideological fact checkers will never have heard of Arnold, so such a statement is probably safe.

Speaking of 'safe' can one now discuss the cheap, non-toxic drugs which were banned for unclear reasons? These included a drug originally used for malaria and which I have prescribed for decades for night cramps. There is the other one which countless Africans took, and about which there is a current lawsuit in India.

The legacy media is full of dread about these variants. To date all have followed standard medical teaching, which is that they mutate to become more infectious but less lethal.

And still the Canadian/ US border remains closed. Why exactly none can tell. Another mystery only understood by a government man. And in Ontario lockdown continues. I suppose the concept of seasonality is beyond a PHJ. Or maybe it is simply to keep the fear going until the fall resurgence.

Q,1. Have you seen the stupidity of these world leaders in England? What a bunch of clowns. Utter hypocrisy playing to the cameras. Trudeau and good old Joe lost their masks at the cocktail party.

Q,2. Millions and millions of masks have been sold. Who owns, or who has an interest in the companies producing them? Maybe that has something to do with mask mandates.

A,1. That might be a reasonable explanation for this continued incomprehensible mask mandate. There certainly is no scientific one. There are rumors of Ottawa political connections in Canada in the mask supply chain.

Q,2. What is with the Indian lawsuit?

A,2. As I understand it, the Indian Bar association is suing an Indian member of WHO who tried to block the use of the drug which cannot be named in that country. The states which used the drug had excellent results and those where it's use was blocked by local governments had many deaths.

June 16

I was with some non-medical people yesterday, unusual since the virus appeared. The group of people I usually interact with through social media are quite knowledgeable, probably in the same bubble, as are most patients. It was a great shock to realize the incredible fear and misinformation in this new group; and these are not stupid people. They were getting their information from the legacy media and believed completely in WHO and the sainted Dr F.

I thought the torrent of misinformation might be over with the US election, which it was to some extent, but the ongoing inexplicable propaganda indicates other factors at work. The CDC has just announced that if you have had the vaccination, then if you are tested, they use a multiplier of 28. If you have not had the vaccine, the multiplier is 40, which is practically guaranteed to show a piece of dead something. So this is utterly biased and clearly completely unethical. At a multiplier of 34, no live virus has been grown, and even at 24+. So what's going on?

If anyone says anything contrary to WHO guidelines, they risk being deplatformed. Thankfully the Indian Bar Association has just laid criminal charges against some members of WHO.

I will just mention 2 of the silly things I saw yesterday with these people. They were wearing face shields. Surgeons, welders, and nails girls use face shields when using power tools to protect their eyes from flying bits. A shield has no effect at all on an aerosol virus. If you are an ICU nurse treating a virus patient coughing in your face, then use a shield, but any other time is just silly.

Similarly all this disinfecting, spraying Lysol on everything, just as they did in the propaganda videos from Wuhan. This virus is not passed by contact, so all this frantic hand washing doesn't help much. I wonder how many people are sick from all these chemicals they are constantly putting on their hands and transferring it to their mouths. And the poor kids, whose job it is to get down and dirty and so develop immunity. All this excessive cleanliness can't be good for them.

Q,1. I saw some studies which showed the drug which cannot be mentioned on youtube or Facebook was used effectively in the early stages of the virus and saved lives. Big tech, big pharma and big media, by disparaging everything Trump promoted, actually killed people.

A,1. I don't know if it is safe to say, but I believe that is what the Indian lawyers are saying as part of their criminal charges. And yes, I do believe that is true.

Q,2. A lady made some insightful comments, but a little too blunt for current sensibilities.

A,2. Madame, I agree completely, but if I even reproduce your comments on the vaccine I will be immediately deplatformed and will lose my medical license

June 21

What is truth? What is science? What is normal, and what is child abuse?

This is not the world I grew up in. I had a senior patient in my clinic today and we were laughing about the Scotland I described in my autobiography 'Have Knife Will Travel'. She reminded me of these carefree days when boys and girls were expected to look after themselves. Maybe we were utterly naive, but we believed in truth, science and progress, that tomorrow would be a better day.

Where has truth gone? Maybe Joseph Goebbels was right that it always was 'the big lie'. There is enough evidence of that, with the New York Times reporter Pulitzer winner, Walter Duranty, who lied about the Soviet Union, and covered up the Holodomor, when 7 million Ukrainians were deliberately starved to death. The misdeeds of the current legacy media and others is just as awful, concealing among other things lifesaving treatments and the origin of the plague.

And science, once that shining light of the West. Duns Scotus and Thomas Aquinas opened the path, and Giordano Bruno gave his life for it. Science is not inevitable. It was crushed in part of the world when the books of Averroes were burned in AD 1,150. Climategate was a similar inflexion point. Emails revealed the Global Warmists were not exactly reporting the truth. And yet, all governments ignored that scandal, and the Warmists simply carried on. If something as egregious and damaging to the public weal as that could be ignored, then concealing the actual science of immunology, virology, and Public Health was simple.

And what is 'normal'? WHO changed the definition of epidemic and pandemic to remove the word 'lethal'. This means that every annual flu outbreak can be labeled an epi or pandemic, and the mechanism is there for another lockdown. So why would anyone start a little business when it can be taken from them with the stroke of a bureaucrat's pen? Why would anyone be self-employed? Let us all work for the state, which can then print more money to pay us. And if we can't buy food, they will dole it out to us.

And what is child abuse? You tell me. Locked up in solitary confinement for a year, not allowed contact with their peers, no school, and forced to wear a mask for no obvious reason, and maybe forced into treatment they don't need and is potentially harmful.

These thoughts are overwhelmingly sad. Thinking Romans must have felt this way for a century before Rome collapsed. Even before the virus I actually wrote a series of novels describing the coming collapse of the West. If interested google the titles. Most are available in audiobooks as well as print. The series is called 'To Slip the Surly Bonds of Earth'. Book one is 'About the Breaking of the Day' and book four is 'Redemption'. In my fiction the West recovers, but will it in real life?

Q,1. I am glad I won't be around to see what happens if the world continues in this direction. I fear for my descendants, but the truly sad fact is that they are growing up into this type of control and accepting it. They won't know anything else.

Q,2. I agree with you and feel bad for my grandchildren.

Q,3. Chin up Hugh. Hitch up your knickers and carry on. The end for everyone else is just a hurdle for a Scot and hope is a side benefit of determination.

A,1. You are right. Man up! This is not like our grandfathers going over the top into the machine guns. Remember Martin Luther, 'here I stand. I can do none other. So help me God.' or the war poets, like Grenfell,

'The blackbird sings to him,
Brother, brother if this be the last song ye shall sing,
Sing it well, for you may not sing another,
Brother sing.'

June 27

Against all scientific evidence lockdown continues in Ontario, Canada. Will it end before the fall resurgence? Well that depends on what the PCR multiplier is. If we ramp up to 45x we can probably find a bit of dead protein here and there, and so continue the charade and keep schools closed. We did manage it last summer, so why not this one?

We have now been given leave to discuss the origins of the virus. Anyone who had the slightest knowledge, knew that it was manufactured. The story of the heroic bat which flew 1,000k to the wet market in Wuhan, while carrying a virus which somehow doesn't infect bats, was always laughable. This propaganda theory published in Lancet, which used to be a reputable medical journal, simply showed that science is no longer science. Lancet has since apologized, but it was such obvious propaganda, that how could anyone take that journal seriously in the future? Sadly I no longer bother to read Canadian general medical journals, as I don't know what is fact or fiction.

For reasons only known to themselves, the sainted Dr and friends, against medical advice and even perhaps federal law, funded this research. Fortunately the virus which escaped or was released was tightly targeted at the ill elderly. But one hears that a SARS virus, which really is deadly, is also a subject of gain of function. Why? To eliminate humanity? Fortunately I had published posts on the origin of the virus last year before it became verboten!

What is worse was the censorship of the repositioned drugs which cannot be named and are still banned in some countries. I saw ridiculous reports of side effects from a drug I have been using for 40 years for night cramps. One cannot but believe that the banning of these drugs will eventually be seen as a tragedy equal to the disastrous legacy of lockdown.

Amazingly I heard that the US funding for the Wuhan lab continues, and that Australia may also be contributing. We know who is funding the research into Anthrax, whose only conceivable purpose is a bioweapon. But who is funding the research into Prions in the leaky lab? Prions produce Mad Cow Disease which is 100% lethal. They are not living so can only be destroyed at a high temperature. So why make them?

Edna Quammie and I had actually decided that they made an excellent bioweapon and had almost completed a book on that before the release of this coronavirus. If interested, Google the title, Prions from Wuhan.

July 4

For over a year the blameless innocent children of Ontario, Canada have been imprisoned by the command of people of uncertain loyalty. Kipling wrote about the tragedy of WW1, especially about the young Australians and New Zealanders in that lunatic Dardanelles exploit.

'They shall not return to us the resolute, the young,
the eager and whole hearted whom we gave.
But the men who left them thriftily to die in their own dung,
shall they come with years and honor to the grave?' Or the men who ordered the 17,000 young Canadian casualties in one battle in 1917.

'I died in Hell.
They called it Passchendaele.'

The last 18 months is this century's equivalent. A war supposedly against a virus, tightly targeted at the unproductive ill elderly. In theory lockdown and all other futile orders were to give granny another 1 month of life. I belong to a group called The Dinosaur Club, the people who worked in the Operating Rooms in Toronto General Hospital in the 70s. If interested, google the book I wrote with my scrub nurse, Edna Quammie, about the wild, glorious, fun filled times in a major hospital following Woodstock. It is called 'The Big House,' and is available in audiobooks. We are definitely the 'at risk' group on the basis of age, but no one has died.

The concept that lockdown would protect us, at the expense of our children, never had any basis in Western medicine. It actually did the opposite. Most of the infections were home based. If it did anything, it slowed the spread of community immunity among the healthy, thus placing grandma at greater risk and encouraging mutations. We have known this since May of 2020, and yet lockdown continues in Ontario. Why?

And all the closures of the Mom and Pop stores and restaurants. Even the dullest Public Health Johnny must have seen the figures that there was no increase in illness in the grocery store clerks. So none of these closures was ever medically justified.

And this PCR test? Well, many people now know that it is, how would you phrase this to avoid the algorithm? Perhaps not something you should bet on. So simply stop doing it, as they have done in Singapore and look at hospitalizations only.

But it is what they have done to the young, especially the children, which is unforgivable. There is a medical condition called 'The Hygiene Hypothesis' which means if you keep the kids too clean, it damages them, making them more liable to allergies, asthma, and the like. And what's happening with all this sanitizer on the kids, which they must inevitably swallow? And this masking which will interfere with facial emotional recognition. And the isolation which will interfere with learning socialization.

I have to be very careful as docs in Canada can lose their license for not parroting the party line. But the whole basis of Western medicine is 'primum non nocere,' first do no harm. God help us all. How will this end? Will these Benedict Arnold's walk away unscathed, or will Justice prevail?

Q,1. What happened to all these military built camps to serve if the hospitals were overloaded?

A,1. None of them were ever used in Canada. Even in the US and the UK at the height of the problem last year only a very few beds were ever occupied, and then they were torn down. A great expense, all for nothing. And then these tent cities were put up in Canada again last winter but were never used. An exercise in poor planning and utter futility. If they were really concerned, then cross train ICU staff during the summer, when there are fewer respiratory cases, equip a couple of wards and mothball them until the next winter. This was never done, anywhere. So obviously no one in authority was actually that concerned.

Q,2. All the MSM in Canada and all the talk show hosts spout the same Fauci line. Who do you listen to?

A.2. I know it is hard to find anything resembling the facts as I know them. I find Sky Australia quite good, and WION, an Indian channel, is not bad. I have found nothing else. It is more a case of looking for names of good docs who appear on some podcasts. An Irish engineer, Ivor Cummins, is an excellent source of accurate information.

July 10

The sky is falling! Again! The almost deadly Delta variant of the virus is upon us. The CDC has reactivated summer mandatory masking. It's déjà vu all over again. And the US/ Canadian border remains closed, for you peons, but not us important chaps.

The new scary Delta variant, or Scariant, as one wicked Irishman calls it, (names will get you censored, as I found out last year when I mentioned the heroine Dr Ai Fen), is actually the renamed Indian variant. This has been the dominant strain in England for months. The Gompertz curve of deaths is unchanged with virtually no deaths in the last few weeks, averaging 25 per day.

There was a recent court case in Portugal where the judge decided, based on the evidence, that the official death figures could be divided by 10. This is roughly what most people have concluded about the CDC figures, which means the actual number who died of the virus, not with, in England is about 2 or 3 in the last few days.

So much for the deadly variant. Sadly for the fear mongers this one can be dumped into the trash can of history along with the Essex, the South African, the Brazilian, and the tooth fairy variant. It remains a fact of life that viruses mutate to infect more people and kill less.

Public health, as a scientific discipline, committed hara-kiri (Japanese ritual disembowelment) when it brought in mandatory universal masking in the middle of last summer when there were virtually no deaths, as people were outside in the sunshine with high Vit D levels. The masks were clearly to keep the fear going and people inside until the falling Vit D levels produced the standard fall resurgence. Obviously this new mask mandate is for the same reason.

The fear drives perfectly healthy people, at no risk to themselves or others, to line up for this PCR test. In Canada the test is run at a CT of 42, which means a tiny piece of protein is magnified a few trillion times. It has been estimated that 97% of positive tests are meaningless. In Frankfurt I hear no test with a CT over 24 is accepted. In Singapore it was 20, and now they have stopped it completely unless the patient is in hospital with a respiratory illness.

Masking adults simply produces fear and paranoia. A recent study surprisingly suggests that children may be physically harmed. We knew it produced psychological damage, but this suggestion of physical harm is new. There is also new data from Australia and New Zealand which suggests that the Hygiene Hypothesis is actually worse than we thought. It was assumed that overprotecting kids from dirt and common diseases would result in the long term in more allergies and autoimmune diseases. The fear was also that their immune systems would not develop properly. The reported significant increase in Respiratory Syncytial Disease in kids seems to confirm our worst fears.

Comparing videos of sporting events with packed, mask less crowds, which have produced no spike in cases, with planes full of sad, silent masked people jammed tightly together, with equally no increase in transmission. I wrote about my experiences as a traveling surgeon teaching joint replacement, in a book called 'Have Knife Will Travel'. Travel then was fun with caviar, cigarettes, and champagne. First they banned caviar and foie gras because of the animal rights people. Then they banned cigarettes. Then we shuffled shoeless through security because of one incompetent shoe-bomber 20 years ago. And now to add to the indignity, we travel faceless, hidden behind a wet soiled mask.

The censors will now allow discussion of the origin of the virus but talk of treatment remains verboten. I understand the money and politics involved with big tech censorship. But in Canada we docs are forbidden to discuss treatment by our own regulatory organization, with the threat of loss of medical license. If I was a young doc looking for research grants, a position in a university, a job in a teaching hospital, or had a young family, I would keep my mouth shut also. This is unheard of in the West. In Cuba, North Korea, China, and the old Soviet Union this was reality. But in Kanada? What is going on?

Sadly I hear that Japan, always one of my favorite sane countries, has given way to pressure, and will allow only a few token spectators at the

Olympics. None of you serfs, just us important government chaps, who are immune to all the ills of life, including viruses.

The only good news is that if this lunacy continues I will have enough posts for the follow-on book to Journal of the Plague Year(2020). This one will be '2021'.

Q,1. I laugh sometimes at your comments, but sadly there is too much truth there. People have known for years that every year the regular flu mutates, so why are they so surprised that this does too? So live with it. Time to get back into the real world.

Q,2. Delta has got to be on the way out and Lambda is coming.

A,1. The mutants will keep coming, especially with a partially effective vaccine, which acts as a driver of mutation. We were warned that widespread use of a non-sterilizing vaccine in the middle of an epidemic, will produce more infective variants. One of the major concerns is that there may eventually be complete viral escape, which means that the virus will be able to avoid not only the induced immunity produced by the vaccination but also all the natural immunity which the body has. Then what? The great extinction?

July 16 at 8:15 PM

Well, well, well! The tragedy is unfolding, and wonder of wonders, it has been reported in a serious newspaper, the Toronto Sun. In Canada in the under 65 age group there were 5,500 deaths attributed to lockdown, and 1,300 who died with or of the virus. Remember the recent trial in Portugal, where the judge decided that the official deaths with the virus, as opposed to of, could be divided by 10. Even in the worst case, the deaths from lockdown were much, much higher than from the virus. Many were due to drugs, especially fentanyl, which also comes from Wuhan.

These figures are not unexpected, as the virus was tightly targeted at the ill elderly, who had significant comorbidities, such as dementia, diabetes, etc. In Sweden most who died were over 80 and had exceeded the average life expectancy. We knew this a year ago, as I pointed out then. And yet the modelers, who guided the Public Health Johnnies, ignored this, producing ludicrous exaggerations, as they did for H1N1, Ebola, Mad Cow Disease, and Global Warming. It is interesting to note that many of the same characters were involved in the H1N1 fiasco. I dutifully lined up for that particular jab. And yet in 2009, when the scandal was broken by the German newspaper Der Spiegel, in spite of the fact that I was crisscrossing the world teaching joint replacement, I knew nothing about it. There were no blaring headlines that I remember.

In spite of current extreme censorship, more facts keep leaking out. We are still not allowed to discuss treatment in social media, and in Canada, docs have been threatened with loss of medical license. I mean, why?

We can now discuss the origin, which began in North. Carolina, where spike protein transfer was developed, and who trained the Bat Lady of Wuhan. When 'gain of function' research was banned in the US, it was moved to Wuhan. That level 4 lab was supposed to be international, but the French, who designed it, were kicked out and replaced by the CCP military. It sounds like a bad novel.

The actual research was done in an adjacent level 2 lab, about as secure as a nails salon. And the rest is history. The lab workers got sick in October 2019. It could have been stopped then, but the brave Chinese docs who tried to warn the world were silenced. In the Chinese Lunar New Year, with the connivance of WHO, the virus was spread all over the world.

Then there were the propaganda videos from China of lockdown, and contrary to all medical teaching, WHO and the CDC, forced it on an unsuspecting world. Why, oh why? There have been in excess of 20 published papers showing lockdown is of no medical value, rather the reverse, and yet 18 months later, it continues in some areas, like Canada. The report in the Toronto Sun, from official government figures, shows what a disaster it was and is. And those figures are only the immediate damage. The economic destruction, the missed medical treatments, and the damage to families and children will play out over the years to come. In other words, the tragedy of this epidemic was not the virus, or even the banning of useful drugs which could have prevented innumerable deaths. It was the lockdown.

My generation has had its day, and a pretty good day it was, as I described in the book I wrote with Edna Quammie, 'The Big House, Toronto General Hospital', describing the wild times in the 70s and 80s. But the outlook for the young looks grim, especially if governments insist on giving them this needle. It makes one think of Augustine, the Bishop of Hippo, surrounded by Vandals destroying everything, looking from North Africa at the lights going out in Rome. "It is finished," he said. And it was. The West descended into darkness for 1,000 years. I so hope that view is wrong.

Q,1. When the eviction moratorium ends in the US, deaths by lockdown are going to skyrocket. If the virus had been allowed to run its course it would just be a bad memory by now. It can't be proved that even one life was saved by lockdown.

A,1. That certainly is what the evidence from Sweden suggests. All the medical evidence points to lockdown as being the main cause of death during this pandemic and will be for years to come.

Q,2. You have verified what a doc friend of mine told me months ago. I believe it was the University of North Carolina at Chapel Hill where Bat Woman was trained to carry out gain of function.

A,2. That is what I understand. But why did the sainted Dr continue to fund her when she returned to Wuhan?

July 22 at 10:50 PM

Riddle me this one. If there was no testing, would anyone know that there was a deadly virus abroad which had shut down the world? Once you finish laughing, let me bore you with some data. Sadly we see the Dunning-Kruger effect in action, as the Public Health Johnnies, the legacy media, and the politicians seem to have difficulties understanding the simplest data.

Anyway, data! 19,000 PCR tests were carried out in Ontario yesterday. Less than 200 were positive, a rate of 0•9%. The problem is that there is a false positive rate of 1%. This means if 2% are positive, half have no trace of virus. What is worse is that a multiplier of 42 is used in Ontario, which means that 97% of the actual positive tests have no illness and only a trace of a coronavirus protein, not necessarily this virus. So they are not sick and they don't transmit.

So what would happen if we stopped testing and got rid of these silly masks? Almost certainly nothing until falling Vit D levels lead to the fall resurgence of respiratory infections.

In Ontario we are being allowed some freedoms, and for that we are grateful. But restrictions continue, in spite of the fact that we have known for more than a year that lockdown has no positive effect on the spread of a highly infectious respiratory virus.

If lockdown affected the virus at all, it encouraged the development of variants, and by delaying community immunity, thus put the vulnerable at increased risk.

The tech giants continue to censor social media, so treatment cannot be discussed. By denigrating possible treatments this stance has likely increased mortality. Obviously this is due to financial and political issues, and while regrettable, is understandable. What is not obvious is why Canadian docs are not allowed to comment on treatment, under threat of loss of medical license.

Giordano Bruno was burned at the stake in 1600 for having the wrong scientific opinion. But then the Enlightenment came, and people were free to express opinions and explore new knowledge, at least in the West. There were episodes of insanity like the Salem Witch Trials in 1692, and of course free speech was suppressed by the Socialists, the National Socialists in Germany and the International Socialists in the Soviet Union and Eastern Europe.

We thought when The Wall came down in 1989, that in most of the civilized world people were free to express opinions.

But working at a university I saw a gradual erosion. It happened so slowly we didn't really recognize it. Looking back we now see it, and I wrote about it with Edna Quammie, my long term scrub nurse, in our book 'The Big House, Toronto General Hospital.1972 to 1984.'

When I came as an immigrant to Toronto in 1972, it was full of bounce and swagger, work like crazy, make money, make love, new inventions, 'the roaring boys bravado.' And then it all seeped away as the administrators and committees took over, the benchwarmers, the has-beens and never-wases.

And now we are all controlled by these gray little bureaucrats, these Adolf Eichmann's, who impose their arbitrary and nonsensical rules. They have destroyed lives and likely irreparably damaged children with this futile lockdown. Ultimately it is what Hannah Arendt described in her book 'The Banality of Evil.'

Q,1. A former surgeon and clinical professor, was fired for supporting informed consent for children being offered the COVID jab. This is so terribly wrong and so utterly sad.

Q,2. Several other people commented on the lack of truly informed consent with this needle.

A,1@2. How can a child, or a teenager, give informed consent, when doctors don't know the short term or worse, long term side effects of the needle? The trial isn't finished.

Q,3. Ontario went down the rabbit hole and unfortunately the clock seems to have stopped ticking. I sit and wonder when we will ever get back to normal, when we are ever going to get our rights back, and when I can I take this effin mask off? The answer seems to be 'never'.

Q,4. If I need a test to tell me I have the virus, then it isn't much of a virus, fake, planned or not.

A,4. What I don't understand is all these people with no symptoms lining up to be tested, knowing if they get a positive test they will have to remain at home for fourteen days. Strange, eh? Is their life outside the home so terrible that they want to stay locked up at home?

Q,5. As you say, institutions get taken over by gray little bureaucrats, who seek political funding and enjoy control.

A,5. As my mother used to say, 'he who pays the piper calls the tune.' So our licensing bodies are the tail wagging the dog, and the dog, the doctors, have no independence.

July 29 at 4:04 PM

Medical clinic quiet today; thinking again of Wilfred Owen, one of the greatest of the War poets,

'Strange friend,' said I, 'here is no cause to mourn.'
'None,' said the other, 'none save the undone years,
the hopelessness.'

I see in the clinic poor kids, achy and obese from lack of exercise, wearing these stupid useless masks, lonely and scared by the lies of the media, trapped at home and unable to travel. The world for us boomers was so different, so wonderful, as I described in my book on the life of a traveling surgeon, 'Have Knife Will Travel'. Other than some vague regrets of missing Japan in Sakura time, the lockdown has had little effect on me. But the poor kids, jailed with no word of parole.

But even for us, essential workers, it is starting to feel that we are the inhabitants of a doomed city with Batu Khan and the Golden Horde of Mongol cavalry on the horizon or sitting beside a dying fire watching the circling wolves. Pessimism I guess, but look at the news, the real news, not that fake stuff peddled by the legacy media, the BBC, CNN, and other sycophants. In Canada the Feds paid them off, and I doubt it is different elsewhere.

Finding real news is so hard. Reputable scientists are canceled. Posts and videos appear and then vanish as the algorithm hunts them down. Docs and scientists are forbidden to discuss treatment. Mere mention of useful, totally safe drugs will produce immediate censoring. What is worse is that in Canada, any discussion on the vaccine may result in removal of license to practice medicine.

Big tech is obviously being paid off, but why elected authorities? What is it that they are desperate to conceal? Something is clearly rotten somewhere.

Our overlords have now given us permission to discuss the origin of the virus. Not that there is much to discuss. The French, who built the lab in Wuhan, warned the US in 2016, before being kicked out in 2017, and being replaced by the CCP military. Knowing this, the sainted Dr continued to fund this 'gain of function' research which was so dangerous it was banned in the US. In other words, US funds were given to develop a bioweapon in a military lab of a hostile nation. What does that sound like to you? Is this Benedict Arnold territory?

We can only be thankful that it was a relatively harmless virus, tightly targeted at the ill elderly. Virtually no healthy person under 60 was at any risk, and yet WHO and the CDC, following the dictat of the Chinese communists, destroyed the world's economies. What will happen when a really bad one comes from that lab?

Lockdown was such an obviously ridiculous concept that one wonders how the Chinese communists managed to convince the world to shoot themselves in the foot. I know they own WHO, and seem to have something on the CDC, and possibly have influence on these ridiculous Global Warmists and virus computer modelers. But why did most Public Health Johnnies go ahead with something, which even the least intelligent had to know, would result in a tsunami of collateral deaths from despair, missed medical treatments, and in the third world, starvation?

And the CDC has just made the ridiculous suggestion of masking forever, with or without the vaccine, even on kids. Makes you think of Shakespeare's Julius Caesar, 'oh judgment thou art fled to brutish beasts, and men have lost their reason.' Or is this simply financial, to keep the fear going to ensure everyone is vaccinated again and again and again?

Q,1. Do you think they are trying to cull as many of us as possible so there will be fewer of us to contend with? They should read The Book of Revelations.

A,1. Hard to believe. That is really 'tin hat' thinking. But, but, but, but a certain billionaire has been talking about too many people.

Q,2. Are drugs which cannot be named banned in Canada?

A,2. It is not safe to mention these drugs by name on social media as it may result in deplatforming. I have not been able to get it in any local drug store. They say they don't have it and won't order it. I have been using Quinine, which is available. It is the more toxic form of the other but as I have been prescribing it for decades for use in leg cramps at night, I think it is perfectly safe. I find it incredible that drugs like these, with a long totally safe history cannot be discussed openly. This is not the world I grew up in.

August 4 at 3:35 PM

It really is Alice in Wonderland time.

'The time has come,' the Walrus said,
'to talk of many things
of shoes and ships and sealing wax
of cabbages and kings
and why the sea is boiling hot
and whether pigs have wings.'

Why did it take the CDC so long to confirm what the Nobel laureate who developed the PCR principle has always said, that this was not a specific test for a virus? It cannot distinguish between the flu and the Wuhan virus. And why did they encourage labs to use a multiplier of over 37, or in Canada 42, when they knew that over 24 it was not possible to culture a live virus? Which means 97% of the positive tests are meaningless.

Why is lockdown still touted by various Public Health Johnnies when we have known for a year that it was not only completely ineffective, but actually put the vulnerable at more risk, encouraged the development of variants, and has been responsible for more deaths than the virus?

Why has only one legacy newspaper, the Toronto Sun, reported on government data which shows how terribly destructive lockdown is?

Why is there still this ridiculous mandatory masking? There is no scientific evidence for it and increasing evidence that it is bad psychologically for children, and may be bad physically.

Why are there still social distancing rules? There is no scientific basis for this. Obviously if someone is coughing and spluttering stay away. But no need to social distance if it is a riot or a demonstration?

Why are mom and pop stores closed and big box stores open?

Why are there virtually no deaths in the tent cities if masking and sanitation are so important? If it made any difference, all these poor, ill, immunocompromised drug addicted homeless in San Francisco should be dead? And why has there been no outbreak in grocery store clerks?

Why are schools closed when they never were in Sweden, and there is no documented case worldwide of a teacher being infected by a pupil?

Why, when it has been known for over a year that kids don't get sick with the virus and they don't transmit, are kids being threatened with a treatment, with potential serious short term side effects and whose long term effects are completely unknown?

Why is there this constant drumbeat of fear porn about the Delta variant, which actually is the Indian variant which has been the dominant strain in the UK for months, with virtually no deaths?

Why is there this frenzy of cleaning with products which may or may not be toxic, when it is known that the virus is not spread by contact?

Why are patients told that there is no outpatient treatment? Wait at home till you turn blue and then go to the hospital.

Why in Canada have docs been threatened with loss of medical license if they discuss treatment with patients?

Why does any mention of drugs, which are totally safe and have been in use for years, result in deplatforming?

The only good news is that judges in Spain and Alberta have struck down some of the most egregious edicts. Who would ever have thought that freedom would depend on lawyers and judges?

Q,1. And why are illegals flooding into the US with no testing while at the same time the Washingtons are screaming like Karen's that we need masks and the jab?

A,1. I admit, it is a little hard to understand that one. The sainted Dr, who has opinions on everything else, for some reason won't comment on that.

Q,2. I see a study from Massachusetts published by the CDC, where 74% of these infected were already vaccinated.

A,2. Yes. The vaccine doesn't stop you from getting infected and transmitting the virus. In many countries the introduction of the vaccine rollout saw a large jump in death rates. There is speculation that people seem especially susceptible and get really sick in the first couple of weeks after the vaccination.

Q,3. The fear of losing one's job or social ostracization seems so widespread. No one is standing up.

A,3. Sadly that is true. But this fear and necessity to conform has been coming for years. The Social Justice Warriors began in the seventies, but we didn't notice them and retreated one inch at a time. We never found a hill to die on. Edna Quammie, my long term scrub nurse, and I finally realized what had been happening when we looked back, while writing our reminiscence for the book called 'The Big House, Toronto General Hospital 1972 to 1984.'

August 11 at 5:27 PM

Welcome to the virus 2-step dance! 1 step forward, 2 steps back.

The step forward was monumental, if ignored by the legacy media and the Public Health Johnnies (PHJs). The CDC has recognized that the PCR test, as currently done, cannot differentiate between the virus and flu. They have also recognized that the cycle threshold (CT) should not be above 24 for post vac patients. Sadly they still allow up to 37 for others, and in Canada a CT of 42, which means 97% of positive tests are meaningless. And yet these tests are still done by the thousands, so someone is making a lot of money.

The big lawsuit in Germany and the US is based on this, that small businesses were bankrupted as a result of this meaningless test, which authorities knew was meaningless.

It is hard not to feel a certain schadenfreude watching Australia and New Zealand tie themselves in knots with repeated lockdowns, trying to keep out a highly infectious low pathogenic virus. There is naturally some resistance to the vaccine, as in these countries more people have died of car accidents than the virus. Even if everyone submits to the vaccine, it won't make much difference as seen in Iceland and Israel. The vaccine doesn't stop the virus. Australia started as a penal colony so maybe they are returning to their roots with their ongoing lockdown.

I do apologize to my Australian friends who probably won't think that is funny.

A patient asked me the other day about treatment. As a simple orthopedic surgeon I of course know nothing about that, and even if I did, in Canada I am not allowed to talk about it. We are told to tell the patient to go home, isolate, and if they turn blue, go to a hospital. I suggested that the patient see a Naturopath, something I never expected to do in my whole life. At least the naturopath can give them useful things.(I have had to remove the names of these products at my publisher's request.) Come to think of it, maybe a vet, as the vet probably has the drug which cannot be named. It really begs the question, if there is no outpatient treatment allowed, why test?

We all know that a virus mutates to infect more people and kill less, and this one is doing just that. J had a good point I had not thought of before. The virus was designed to readily infect humans, so it doesn't have to mutate much to get more infectious, so there is a far less risk of it making a mistake and turning deadly.

I knew nothing about the H1N1 scandal in 2009. It is remarkably similar to this one. Big tech hasn't realized that so the information is still there, so look it up before it disappears. Many of the players are the same. It was for that outbreak the definitions were changed removing the word 'lethal', so any bad flu year can now be called a pandemic. It was a German newspaper Der Spiegel, who blew the whistle on that one, pointing out that while there were lots of positive tests, there were no sick people, and the vaccine wasn't that safe. Interestingly I just saw a video from another German newspaper Der Bild, blowing the whistle on this one, but I can't find it now.

I just heard on the car radio, that in the run up to the re-election of our dear leader in Canada, those who have doubts about the vaccine are going to be in worse trouble than those in increasingly totalitarian France. Who knows! Maybe it's only political posturing. But if the Dear Leader implements his threat, then 'pray for us now in hour of our darkness.'

Q,1. I have a friend who is fully vaccinated and he just tested positive for the virus. Why he would get tested when he had no symptoms is difficult to understand. The CDC has just said that the PCR test is worthless anyway.

A,1. I have been saying for over a year that the PCR test run at over a 24CT is meaningless. The CDC has just said it can't differentiate from a cold or the flu. So why, oh why are we still doing it by the thousands. Who is making money from this worthless endeavor?

Q,2. Been saying this for over a year, but no one is listening.

A,2. The serious scientists and docs, who have pointed all this out, are silenced by their employers, associations, or by big tech. But why? Money or the great reset?

August 16 at 5:12 PM

'Out of the mouth of babes and suckings thou hast ordained truth.' Psalms(8:2). Never more true than now.

I had a young woman who works in Tim Horton's in my medical clinic today. Tim's is a famous Canadian coffee chain. She was deeply unimpressed with this overhyped deadly virus. Someone wanted to vaccinate her son, and she was furious. She pointed out that she, and all the other girls in Tim's, had been exposed to all comers throughout the whole plague, and none had been ill. She pointed out that none of the grocery store clerks that she knows got sick. One of her friends did get the virus and got better in a week with no treatment. And for this they want to vaccinate her kid!

I only wish that this young lady was running Public Health Canada. She clearly has a better understanding than these gold plated, indexed pensioned, no nothings and their utterly incompetent computer modelers.

An hour later I had in a young lady from the Congo, who has been working as a grocery store clerk since she got to Canada. She said no one in her store had been sick. She was also furious because her young son, who has a basketball scholarship to a US university, has been forced to take the vaccine. I sympathized with her as my young son has also been forced to take it in order to return to in-person learning at his university.

As a medical student I spent several months in Warsaw in 1963, in the height of communism, or as close to communism as any true Pole would accept. These were the people after all who whipped the Red Army at the battle of the Pripet Marshes. I really don't remember that the docs had any particular restrictions, other than of course equipment, as any socialist state is going to produce shortages in very short order. It is after all, a well-known statement, that if the socialists were running the Sahara desert in a few weeks there would be a shortage of sand.

This is the first time in the West doctors are forbidden to prescribe drugs which have a long successful track record, for no clear reason. Even mentioning them by name will result in censorship by social media. In Canada it is even worse, as docs have been threatened with loss of medical license if they don't follow exactly the edicts of the utterly corrupt WHO and the very questionable CDC. So do docs in Canada currently have more restrictions than the docs in Poland in the height of communism?

The results from Iceland and Israel, the most vaccinated countries in the world, are not promising. Our Dear Leader in Canada is ordering millions more doses of the vaccine. Eh? A booster? Every six months? And no discussion is allowed? 2 years ago who would have thought that discussion would be banned? That this tightly targeted virus could effectively end freedom in the Western world?

But then, on reflection, of course we knew that we were approaching the edge of the abyss. I wrote about it in my book 'Have Knife Will Travel'. In the seventies, I and my engineering colleague developed the current method of fixing artificial joints in place before the useless FDA began to regulate implants. If we were starting now, it is unlikely we could ever have done it, given the regulations and restrictions set up by bureaucrats and administrators. That must be true in most other fields.

And it's not just medicine. Look at the disaster in Afghanistan. As a child of the British empire, I knew the history of that part of the world. Clearly the US Foreign Office did not. It is called the graveyard of empires, Alexander the Great, the Genghis Khan, the British and the Russians, all conquered and all left, and it was as if they had never been. Nothing has changed in 2,000 years, nor is it ever likely. Nation building? Give your head a shake!

Q,1. The entire globe has been a battlefield forever. History is replete with war after war. Will it ever end?

A,1. I think not. All empires get complacent, corrupt, and then collapse. And then barbarians stroll over the undefended walls. The saying is well known. Bad times produce strong men. Strong men produce good times. Good times produce weak men. Weak men produce bad times. Camille Paglia writes that art is very reflective of what is happening and it is possible to judge the condition of a civilization by its art. As our current symbol of art is a toilet, or a crucifix in a bowl of urine, sadly Camille may be right.

August 20 at 5:25 PM

'The hand of the reaper takes the ears that are hoary,

but the voice of the weeper wails manhood in glory.' Death is part of life. We all walk through that gate sooner or later. As Adam Smith wrote that 'death is that quiet harbor after the turbulent seas of life.' For we elderly, maybe we look forward with equanimity, but not for our children. For them, as Dylan Thomas wrote

'Do not go gently into that good night,

but rage, rage against the dying of the light.'

And yet for the last disastrous 18 months, and for the foreseeable future, we are sacrificing our children. They are being asked to put their lives on hold in the mistaken belief that the ill elderly will live another 2 months. Not only has the lockdown not saved granny, but no one asked us seniors if we were prepared to ask the young to pour down the drain, 'the sweet red wine of youth.'

Most people now know how fudged the official figures are. Roughly about 90% of deaths were with the virus, and 10% due solely to it. But even the utterly suspect government figures are beginning to show that far more people died as a result of the lockdown than from the virus. In Sweden the average age of death was over 80, older than the average life expectancy.

So the young have been asked, or ordered, to sacrifice themselves for nothing. The evidence is, that if lockdown did anything at all, it encouraged the development of variants and slowed community immunity, as we will see in the fall resurgence.

For kids it has been a disaster. These poor masked tiny things who have not learned to read human faces. The lunacy of kids in sports running wearing a mask. Even the dullest Public Health Johnnies and even the sainted Dr, who admitted privately that universal masking was silly, must surely feel some guilt. But they are bureaucrats, being doctors in name only, so maybe they simply don't care.

'We are all in this together' the politicians chant. But we are not. It is the young, and the lower middle and working class who have paid the price with their jobs, their health, and their emotional well-being. The small businessmen have lost everything, their life savings, their businesses and soon their houses. And wait for the inflation to come. The best indicator of inflation is the grocery store. In Canada the prices seem to have doubled, which means our dollar is worth about 50 cents and falling rapidly.

Unbelievably, we are still forbidden to talk about treatment. The policy is still go home, isolate, and when you turn blue go to a hospital. Outpatient treatment is largely forbidden. This is the first time in history that effective treatments have been denied. The health care system in Canada and the UK is in shambles, and we are entering fall, when a reduced Vit D will lead to a virus resurgence.

The incompetence demonstrated at the highest levels among politicians, Public Health Johnnies, WHO and the CDC is such that it is hard to accept stupidity as the sole reason. But it is equally hard to postulate an ulterior motive. Recent events show that this incompetence extends to the military.

The British disastrous retreat from Kabul in 1842, was led by general Elphy Bey (google the name), a dithering incompetent, a disgrace! The current retreat from Kabul matches the British for sheer incompetence. I guess the current head General was too busy being woke to read military history. I always thought that the generals in WW1 were terrible, but this new crop clearly comes from the same mold.

Q,1. The current leaders of the West combine vanity with the attention span of a gnat with the expected result.

A,1. Sadly, Dunning-Kruger strikes again, and their back-ups are subject to the Peter Principle, that bureaucrats are promoted to the level of their incompetence.

August 24 at 3:18 PM

Let us start with something which is not controversial. People with no symptoms do not transmit the virus in sufficient quantities to infect others. So, if you are sick, stay at home. If you are not there is no need for testing, masking, social distancing, or lockdown.

The number of absolutely healthy children in the US who have died of the virus is vanishingly small, and kids don't transmit. We have known this for over a year. I am still waiting to hear of a documented case of a pupil infecting a teacher. The infection rate in teachers in Sweden, where schools for the young never closed, was less than other professions. So open schools with no testing, no masking, no silly plexiglass, and no distancing.

We thought that the hepa-filters on planes explained the absence of infection. It turns out that hepa-filters have no effect on an airborne virus, so schools don't need to retrofit. I guess sick people don't fly. Let's not kid-on that these dumb masks on planes do anything.

But what more can we say? We all like to think of ourselves as Childe Roland,

'And in a flash of flame I saw them and I knew them all.
And yet, dauntless the slug-horn to my lips I set and blew,
Childe Roland to the Dark Tower came.'

People wonder why so few docs and scientists have spoken out about the obvious foolishness in the handling of the virus. The same has been true for the last 30 years about global warming. There are very few Childe Rowlands, and while there are not that many Giordano Bruno's, who was burned at the stake in 1600, for expressing a contrary view of science, we still have a lot to lose.

The book 'The Gulag Archipelago', which exposed the horrors of socialism, would not have been written if Aleksandr Solzhenitsyn had not privately complained about the equipment the Red Army had when fighting the Germans. For this he ended up in the gulag. Milan Kundera's 'The Joke' was written in the sixties describing the consequences of telling a joke in Eastern Europe. Our equivalent is Cancel Culture. The consequences for a young doc or scientist speaking out is pretty brutal. They will lose their job, research grants, and any possibility of promotion. In Canada it is worse, as we have been threatened in writing with loss of medical license if we don't follow the party line. If they have a family with kids, who is going to take that risk? If you think you would be different, read Christopher Browning's book 'Ordinary Men.' You will note that those who do speak out, as in the great global warming fiasco, have gray hair, and are frequently retired.

Free speech is no longer free and can be silenced easily by social media. So we have to self-censor. Last year, as many of my posts were disappearing, I published them in book form. Google Journal of the Plague Year(2020). As the lunacy continues, in another 4 months I can publish 2021. So please help me by adding your comments and thoughts as I can publish these too, albeit incognito.

Saying anything about the vaccine is verboten, so let's call it the needle, to avoid the algorithm.

The results from Israel, the most needled country, shows that whatever immunity there is from the needle is short lived, and the infections are flaring up again. So the needle doesn't stop the disease or the transmission. Countries like Canada are buying millions more needles. This is all playing out as some feared. No one knows if the toxicity of the boosters will go up and the benefits dramatically down. It certainly shows that needle passports have nothing to do with safety or a virus.

Looking around the world, the countries which seem to have done best are those who ignored WHO, the CDC, and the sainted Dr. Those who did worst followed them. New Zealand and Australia are in perpetual lockdown, and with the fall resurgence a month or so away, so will Canada. What will happen when they have used all the borrowed money and the lender wants to collect?

Ah well, it could be worse I suppose. So read the Rubaiyat,

'Ah make the most of what we yet may spend
before we too into the dust descend.'

ADDENDUM

People have been asking about the book, 'Ordinary Men.' It was about Police Battalion 101, a bunch of ordinary German policemen, who ended up committing some of the worst genocidal acts in Poland in WW11.

Q,1. People keep lining up for the needle because the government tells them that if they do, everything will return to normal. But alas this is not the case. Now they want vaccine passports for a vaccine which doesn't stop infection or transmission.

A,1. Exactly. Why do people with no symptoms line up to be tested? Where has sanity gone? Why are we constantly being lied to? Where will it end? Is this the Weimar Republic mark 11?

August 28 at 11:24 AM

Those who thought that big tech censorship would end after the US election were wrong. It is getting worse, not better. In Canada docs can now lose their medical license for not following the party propaganda. What information is so bad it can't be discussed? What must remain hidden? Why can't we name the useful drugs which have been safely used for decades?

For fear of the fierce algorithm let us call that thing injected into your arm the needle.

Everyone, even the despicable legacy media, now admits that the needle doesn't prevent infection and doesn't prevent transmission. Possibly it reduces mortality a little, but only time will tell.

So if the needle doesn't stop infection or transmission then what is this demand for needle passports? The passport tells authorities that someone has had the needle. But so what? They can still get sick, and more importantly, transmit. So what is the passport for? It doesn't mean you are safe. It means nothing. Even the dumbest Public Health Johnny must know this. So why are they pushing this? Why is this an election campaign issue for our Dear Leader in Canada?

And why are kids being forced to take the needle? I had a father and his big tough young son in my clinic yesterday. This big fit young boy has been given an athletic scholarship at a Canadian university, an unusual thing, so he must be extremely good. They are not stupid people and they adamantly don't want the needle. They point out that he is at no risk from the virus and some risk from the needle. The cost /benefit analysis is clear. I completely agreed with them but could not help them. My own young son was forced by his despicable university to take the needle. He looks OK, but we won't really know that for another decade or so.

Hospitals are doing the same, forcing staff who worked through the initial crisis with little or no protection, to take the needle. Makes you wonder why so many Health Care staff remain un-needled, and why some are prepared to walk away from their jobs rather than submit to the needle. Could be they know something?

What is worse is that the sainted Dr, the CDC, and their Public Health lackeys are demanding that people who have recovered from the virus get the needle in order to get the needle passport. It is medicine 101 that after recovery from a virus you have immunity. And yet the sainted Dr is insisting that these people put themselves at risk for no benefit in order to get the needle passport. What sense does this make?

The FDA has just announced that one needle is safe and effective. But how can this be as the trial actually doesn't end for another year or so? Faucian logic? When I wrote my book 'Have Knife Will Travel' about how we developed modern artificial hips and knees, some reviewers did not like it that I clearly loathed the FDA and other similar government bodies. Now I think most people know why.

Having worked with universities and government bodies for years, I always knew, and now I think most people do also, that the worst thing you can hear is, 'I am from the government and I am here to help you.'

Q,1. I can't help but think "Faustian bargain' when a certain doctor's name is mentioned.

A,1. I live in hope. If you know what happened to Dr Faustus in Kit Marlowe's play, then that is what should happen to this guy. The devils came to drag him down to hell. And I hope that they take some of his accomplices with them.

Q,2. Israel is reporting those with the needle are at a higher risk of infection.

A,2. I don't know yet if it is higher, which is what K warned might happen. But it is certainly not stopping infection or transmission, so what's with the needle passport?

September 3 at 5:15 PM

Rejoice! Light at the end of the tunnel. I do hope that it is not an approaching train. The data from Israel cannot be denied. The needle (We can't call it by its real name for fear of censorship.) doesn't stop infection or transmission of the virus.

Moves were afoot to force little kids to take the needle, regardless of the risk, because they might infect granny. The fact that this was never true was being ignored. Kids were never at risk from the virus and they did not transmit.

The Israeli figures show that the needle doesn't stop infection or transmission. This means that there is no justification whatsoever for needling kids. Or for that matter university students, who equally are at no risk, or indeed anyone under 60 who is healthy. So there is no justification for mandatory needling of anyone. The sainted Dr F and his cronies can be told to go and peddle their misinformation elsewhere.

Equally the Israeli figures put an end to the 'Collective' dream of a needle passport. If you can be needled and still transmit the virus, then what exactly is the needle passport telling anyone? Clearly it has nothing to do with safety.

The legacy media is showing it's true colors by refusing to publicize the huge anti-lockdown protests which are occurring worldwide. Sadly the police in many countries are behaving abominably in response to these protests. I never thought I would say that, as decades ago I was the orthopedic surgeon who looked after the police in downtown Toronto. I counted many among them as my friends, as I recounted in my book 'Have Knife Will Travel'. Have things changed or is it simply a few bad apples?

At the end of most medical clinics I feel happy as I interact with so many admirable people bearing up under adversity. But today was depressing. I came to Canada in 1972, in the last immigrant boat from Europe. It was full of kids in their 20s, out to eat the world alive, seeking fame and fortune. It was just after Woodstock, which occurred in the middle of a severe flu epidemic, which everyone ignored. We feel sorry for the poor young people of today struggling with the fear of 'me too-ism.' They will never know the freedom their grandparents had.

What was depressing about today's clinic was for the first time I saw people giving up on Canada. There were always some losers who went home, but today was different. One was a successful woman with a 3 year old child. Schools have been closed here for 18 months. She is so fed up with the incompetence of the various levels of government that she is going back to Brazil which she thinks is doing much better. Another was a successful woman who has been in Canada for 20 years. She can see runaway inflation coming due to the reckless spending and thinks Hungary will be a better place to weather the storm. To see people like that leaving is frightening. I keep telling my son to improve his Mandarin as it looks to me that Singapore is one of the few well managed countries.

In the midst of all this angst there is something wonderful. 2 senior FDA officials have resigned in protest at the Feds pressure to legalize something with inadequate testing. Hard to believe a bureaucrat with integrity exists. Now if only those responsible for the catastrophe of the handling of the virus and the retreat from Kabul would do the same. But sadly, don't hold your breath. Equally sadly, the FDA went ahead anyway, in spite of the resignations.

Q,1. So many of my friends are frantic that they are losing their jobs because they don't want the needle for a variety of reasons. It is tragic and so unnecessary.

A,1. I sympathize. This is grotesque. His university forced my young son to take the needle. He didn't want to but had no choice. Why are they doing this, is it stupidity, cupidity, or collusion?

Q,2. I have just returned for 2 months in Europe. Kids were active and competing in sports. This is like coming back to a police state.

A,2. The tragedy is that the sainted Dr and his lackeys, the PHJS in Canada, must know that kids do not get seriously ill with this virus and they don't transmit. So how can they justify this psychopathic treatment of children?

September 8 at 10:40 PM

We live in fear. What an admission in the West. Cuba, China and North Korea you can understand, but Canada! Since when? Since the virus. Canadian docs have been threatened with loss of medical license if they don't follow the party line. Docs have lost their jobs for disagreeing with the edicts of WHO and the sainted Dr and his cronies.

This is a new and disturbing world. Can you trust your doc to give you an honest opinion? Maybe, if the office door is closed and he has known you for decades. I had some people in my office this morning for rechecks of joints I had done years and years ago. They were telling me how difficult it is to access face to face their GPs. These people are my generation and like me, are not so good with the electronic world. I hear the same complaints from UK patients. I don't know about the US.

There is also the fear of the Cancel Culture. For a long time big tech would de-platform anyone who talked about the origin of the virus. Everyone knew it was made in the lab in Wuhan, funded by the sainted Dr. They kept hidden the real fear that Bat Woman had added HIV stolen from the lab in Winnipeg to the virus she had made in 2018 or earlier. It was May of 2020 before the Koreans decided that if she had, it was inactive so immunity was possible.

Why this subject was verboten was never clear. Was it to smother the evidence that the sainted Dr F and the NIH were involved? The 'bought and paid for' legacy media went along with this coverup.

Patients in Canada who have been told they have the virus are told to go home and when they turn blue go to a hospital. When they ask me about treatment, I tell them I know bad backs and bad knees but very little else. I don't know what to say. So I tell them about the importance of Vit

D, although unbelievably our Canadian federal minister of Health says that's not important. I tell them about simple over the counter agents. (The publisher feels they cannot be named.) But I cannot mention the drugs widely used by the rest of the world. They are not available in Canada in any case, except through your local vet. This is really hard to believe.

And then there is the needle. All sorts of organizations are making it mandatory. There is a looming shortage of health care providers who are walking away rather than accept the needle. And these are the heroic frontline people who worked through the epidemic, initially completely unprotected. Ask yourself, why are these people walking away?

There are huge demonstrations worldwide about the needle and the needle passport. But they are being ignored by the legacy media in every country. So big demonstrations are like throwing a stone into a pond; a big splash and then nothing.

I have to be so careful writing about the needle. I hear one from China is more traditional. It likely doesn't work but seems to have fewer side effects. I hear a safer one is coming, but who knows anything for certain. I don't, and I have no idea when I will.

ADDENDUM

This post was very interesting. Reportedly, very few people looked at it. I eventually realized I had crossed the line and mentioned some of the useful non-prescription medicines in the treatment of this disease. I think this is what is called shadow banning. Since then I have carefully avoided mentioning any treatments.

September 10 at 5:39 PM

I saw a discarded child's mask today, the harbinger of doom. As Newbolt wrote,

'There's a far bell ringing at the setting of the sun
and a phantom voice is singing of the great days done.'

That mask and the fall of Kabul brings to mind the fall of Rome.

As a child I mourned the fall of Rome. The history of my own country, Scotland, like Japan and any other poor mountain state, was constant war, with not much to show for it. Even the loss of the British Empire didn't mean much to me as it was so short lived and the politicians involved in its demise seemed such dreary losers. But Rome, in all its magnificence, to know that it's collapse resulted in 1,000 years of ignorance and barbarism, that was a tragedy.

Since the end of WW11, we have had Pax Americana protecting the world from the horrors of socialism. Maybe the last leader was the last flicker of hope. Like Belisarius, who reconquered the Western Roman Empire for a time and was rewarded by being blinded and forced to beg on the streets of Constantinople. But now, all around us, we see collapse. As Kipling wrote,

'Far called our navies melt away,
on dune and headland sinks the fire.
Lo, all our pomp of yesterday
is one with Nineveh and Tyre.'

The poetry of the past shows the cycles of history. As Yeats wrote,

'Things fall apart, the centre cannot hold
mere anarchy is loosed upon the world.
The best lack all conviction,

while the worst are full of passionate intensity.
The darkness drops again.'

All around we see this collapse, especially the Anglo-sphere. In Australia they are building gulags, sorry, quarantine camps. Chinese Communist Social Credit Scores are appearing everywhere, masquerading as needle passports. As the data from Israel clearly shows, the needle doesn't stop acquiring or transmitting the virus, so a passport serves no medical purpose.

What brought on this melancholy was seeing this tiny, discarded face mask at the clinic door this morning. The masking of children never had any scientific basis, as children do not get sick with this virus and they don't transmit. Everyone has known this for over a year.

Common-sense indicates that a child must be able to see faces to learn how to react to moods. We know that if a child is not socialized early in life there may be major irreversible behavioral problems. Wearing a wet, soiled mask all day cannot be good physically, and there is some recent data showing potential harm.

And where does this frantic push to needle children come from? The cost/ benefit is obviously negative. If it is done purely for money, that is a shocking indictment on our current society. I suppose I should not be shocked given the utter, probably purposeful, failure of Western education. We are producing graduates with little skills or learning. Uber driver or barista I suppose, or even worse HR, who are destroying companies from within. 'Go woke, go broke!' is not just a slogan.

But enough with the sorrow! One of my recent clinical fellows, who returned to England, has just published a major new technical book on Knee Replacement. I was honored to write a chapter for him. It is great to watch the young guys stepping up, the changing of the guard. As John McCrae wrote

'To you we fling the torch
be yours to hold it high.'

So I guess we carry on, one day at a time.

Q,1. I just saw the police confiscating alcohol in Australia. During lockdown the amount per day is rationed by the government.

A,1. Justine, the Dear Leader of Canada and Prince of Woke must be salivating at potentially having such control over his subjects

Q,2. One day at a time! We failed with that long ago.

A,2. I know, mea culpa, I know. Is this Gotterdammerung, the Twilight of the Gods? It makes one think of T.S. Elliot,

'This valley of dying stars,
This hollow valley.
This broken jaw of our lost kingdom.
This is the way the world ends
Not with a bang, but a whimper.'

September 15 at 4:07 PM

I just read something so clever and so funny that it has to be repeated. 'The protected need to be protected from the unprotected by forcing the unprotected to use the protection that didn't protect the protected.' This is the ultimate epitaph of the vaccine, Faucian logic at its finest, true Orwellian doublethink. It is so clever I feel a bit like Oscar Wilde, who when he heard a clever bon mot, said, "I wish I had said that." A friend said, "you will Oscar, some day you will."

Driving downtown to the hospital this morning. Toronto is back, the worst traffic in North America. The schools are finally open after 18 months. True to form, the city-maintenance has every main artery to downtown partly blocked, but no one is actually working. Ah well, at least one form of child abuse is temporarily over and the kids are back in class.

I am sure it does them good emotionally. But the so-called distance learning allowed many parents to hear what their kids were actually being taught. The lies and hatred spewing from some teachers and some curricula has driven some parents ballistic. Their genuine and vociferous complaints can be heard all over the net.

My own kids were taught no history, which I found appalling. If you don't know history you don't know the world, like the guy currently running the US military. It sounds like a tin-hat theory, but if kids are deliberately not taught history it is easy to conceal the horrors of socialism, the Holodomor, the Killing Fields, the Great Leap Forwards, or as they call it in China, the Great Hunger.

Sitting in traffic I turned on the car radio. How silly of me! The announcer, a well-known 'The Science is settled' chap, was busy telling his audience that the information from Israel about the failure of the needle to prevent infection or transmission, was debunked. Why tell such a silly lie when everyone who has access to the net can find in seconds that it is a lie?

And then the same chap interviews some Canadian doc who claims that in her hospital there are many ill patients dying of the virus. I checked the official government stats. No one died yesterday and the weekly average is 2. Was she really a doc? Does anyone ever fact check?

She then said that 10% of patients get 'long COVID'. I think it exists, as it does with all virus infections. Several years ago I got Guillain-Barre after a mild respiratory illness. But it is no more common with this virus than after the flu.

Mea culpa! I have to confess that I failed my Martin Luther moment. After nailing his theses to the church door in Wittenberg, when they came after him, he said, 'here I stand. I can do none other. So help me God.' My university and hospital threatened me with job loss unless I took the needle. University position I don't care, but the hospital I do, so I bowed before the bureaucrats, kissed their feet, and took the needle.

So many health care workers, braver than I, are defying them and walking away. Already I hear a maternity Unit in one hospital has closed as the staff have quit over the mandatory needle. Wait until the winter resurgence and there is no hospital staff. Will the politicians and bureaucrats do the nursing? This will certainly give them an excuse to declare an emergency.

Once you take the first step down to Gehenna there's no end, the 2nd needle, then as in Israel, the 3rd, then the 4th, and on and on. Just as K predicted. He suggested that this might be the answer to the Fermi paradox. Fermi, looking up at the night sky and the billions of stars, asked, 'where is everyone?' I always thought we might nuke ourselves out of existence. Instead of Ragnarök, the battle at the end of time, maybe it will be the needle which eliminates the human race.

I do so hope K is wrong.

Q,1. That quotation needs no explanation in its silliness and yet sad truth. The road ahead grows longer and darker and we may become lost eventually. As an optimist I like to think there is light somewhere, just waiting for someone to throw the switch.

A,1. Where is Octavian, William Tell, Jan Sobienski, or Miltiades when you need him?

September 19 at 6:33 PM

The educated classes are not educated! That idea came to me while listening to a podcast from a brilliant historian and geographer. It was embarrassing to look at the so-called leaders of the Free World posturing during the recent G7 meeting. It was like watching a clown show. They were wearing useless face masks on an empty sunny beach and doing elbow bumps. A charade for us peasants. Even these people must know that the chances of virus transmission under such circumstances is virtually zero.

And an hour later at a cocktail party, no masks, no distancing, and embracing each other.

It is the same with all these mandates. The needle for thee but not if you work in Washington. For John Doe, the needle or else!

Nurses, cleaners, and other hospital staff who worked, with no complaints and no protection through the first wave of the epidemic, are now being disparaged by the legacy media and the politicians. In the spring of 2020, when we all thought this was real and we would die, the retired nurses heard the call of duty and flooded back to work. As I wrote in my book Journal of the Plague Year(2020), describing that time of fear, the camaraderie was uplifting. 'The old warhorses growing young amid the trumpets of battle'.

And now these people, who lived through the worst of the epidemic, who went unprotected into battle because in Canada our Dear Leader had shipped tons of PPE to China in February; these people are being told to submit to the needle or be fired. Where is the gratitude and humanity? No wonder so many are walking away in disgust.

You can't run a health care system without nurses, porters, cleaners, and technicians. If they are not there the system will collapse. How many beds will have to be closed this winter because of this foolish mandate?

As a Canadian doc I am not allowed to write or speak about treatment of the virus or the needle. But not only Canada. In a recent post I dared to mention some simple over-the-counter remedies which I myself use. That post had a tiny percentage of the normal visits. Obviously I was not outspoken enough for a complete ban, but this was a warning to stay away, and keep my mouth shut.

The utter mismanagement of the retreat from Kabul is a clear indication of the collapse of the West. The 70s and 80s were so great, wild, and free, as Edna Quammie and I wrote in our book of reminiscences, 'The Big House'. We failed to recognize the slow decline, with the rise of the little gray bureaucrat and the semi-literate utterly worthless university professors.

Empires rise on hobnail boots and fall in satin slippers. But slippers are more comfortable than boots if you can tolerate the ineffable sadness of watching it all slip away and the coming Dark Ages of poverty, misery, and oppression. As Newbolt wrote, looking at the collapsing British empire,

'there's a far bell ringing at the setting of the sun
and a phantom voice is singing of the great days done.'

I guess in a sense we are all Boethius, who wrote from his prison cell in AD 524, that 'the greatest tragedy is to have been happy once.' At least the young will be spared that. For them, there will be no glad memories.

Ah, lighten up! My wife's lump is not cancer; I have survived the first mandatory needle with no neurological deficits other than some muscle spasms; my kid is doing well in school; the publisher has accepted our most recent book, and my coauthor, Edna Quammie and I have just begun a new one.

Non Nobis Domine!

Q,1. There has been so much misinformation about this Plandemic. Like many people I have been out working every day since this started without taking any excess precautions. I never got sick. Within three days of the second needle there have been three people in my quite small group who have become sick, one requiring airlift to a major hospital for his myocarditis.

A,1. It certainly seems very risky, especially for young men. There is absolutely no information on the fertility of young women. I was hoping to put off having the needle until the adverse effects were so well known that they could no longer force it on people.

Q,2. K and G have given interviews laying out a frightening scenario. That the vaccinated will need boosters upon boosters upon boosters until finally nothing works.

A,2. So far everything these two men have predicted has come true. So maybe this will turn out to be the extinction. Hard to contemplate. The end of the human race thanks to the sainted Dr and the Wuhan lab.

September 24 at 6:24 PM

Riddle me this one. The US northern border is still closed unless you fly across with effectively a needle passport. The southern border is wide open with essentially no checks. So this is about a virus? Thousands of elderly Canadians, the snowbirds, will not be in Florida this winter, an obvious blow to the economy. Is this a punishment for that state's exemplary handling of the virus? Just asking.

Another riddle. Lockdown was never ever considered anywhere, anytime, until Wuhan. In the Black Death, with a roughly 30% mortality, sick people were quarantined, but never healthy. Amazingly the world bought this CCP Ponzi scheme. It was initially trumpeted by that embarrassing WHO chap, who doesn't understand a Gompertz curve, and who during a video interview had never heard of Taiwan.

The selling of this misinformation was helped along by the computer modelers, who have always been just as dramatically wrong as their global warming buddies. What is difficult to understand is why virtually all Public Health Johnnies, with the exception of Sweden, bought into this ludicrous concept.

Eventually even the totally corrupt WHO were so embarrassed, that almost a year ago they pointed out that lockdown was a catastrophic failure, leading to an unimaginable number of collateral deaths. Lockdown had no effect on the infection curves in any country. Some official government figures, like those published in the Toronto Sun, already show that deaths from lockdown far exceed the grossly inflated virus deaths. And yet the lockdown continues? Why?

One constant theme was to 'save' health care systems. But nothing was done last summer or for that matter, this summer, when hospitals were empty, to cross train staff and equip more ICU units. ICU beds are so expensive that they run almost all year at about 90% capacity. Even in the soft summer, elective operations on those who will need an ICU bed after surgery are always being deferred. At a pinch ICUs can run at 120% capacity, so being 'almost full' is an everyday affair.

So what will happen during this resurgence? We already know. Nurses and other staff who worked through the epidemic, with virtually no protection, are being offered the choice of mandatory needle or losing their jobs. An amazing number are choosing to walk away. Since these are the people who know most about the virus and the needle, one wonders why. So will understaffed ICUs be overwhelmed this winter? Eh? Just asking.

It is bitterly amusing that the Quebec government, a staunch proponent of mandatory this and that, have announced a signing bonus of $15,000+ for nurses to remain or to move from part to full time work. I am sure the rest of Canada will soon follow, as will some states in the US. And wait for the signing bonus for nursing home staff.

Future historians will look back on this worldwide lockdown as insanity. And even more tragically this desperate desire to needle kids. If there is no demonstrable benefit, then should you ever accept any cost?

But in the midst of this tragic slaughterhouse of people's lives and dreams, maybe there is some hope. A few European countries are starting to wake up and reject this miasma of fear and misinformation. As the lyrics say,

'we chase the rainbow through the rain,
and hope the promise is not vain,
that morn shall tearless be.'

Q,1. They announce the COVID deaths daily on TV. But why only COVID. How many people die from cancer, car crashes and suicide? Is this just to produce fear?

A,1. And what is worse, we have really no idea how many died with or of the virus. In Portugal a judge ruled in a trial that government deaths from the virus could be divided by ten. In the US we think it is closer to reality if the overall claimed COVID deaths are divided by 17x.

Q,2 'Something wicked this way comes.'

A,2, But is it stalking or blundering along?

Q,3. I rather think the former Doc.

A,3. I know, but I don't like to think that.

Q,4. I have a curious question. The Police Union here in Ontario have said 'no', to the vaccine passport. So if a police officer goes into a Tim Hortons (a major Canadian coffee shop chain) will he/ she be asked for their vaccine passport? If they are served, will the shop be charged with serving our boys/girls in blue if they serve those who don't have the needle?

A,4. That fiasco scenario shows the basic hypocrisy of this craziness. The needle passport doesn't indicate that the bearer is immune to the virus or can't transmit it.

October 1 at 7:56 PM

70,000 health care providers are being laid off in New York. These are the people who put it all on the line, working initially with no PPE, exposed to an unknown and potentially lethal virus. Remember that 70+ unprotected docs in Northern Italy died from that initial blast of virus. Those health care providers who survived either were infected with the virus and recovered or had natural inbuilt immunity. As Housman wrote,

'their shoulders held the sky suspended
they stood, and Earth's foundations stay.
What God abandoned these defended.'

These people survived. Forget this ridiculous idiotic Faucian nonsense of no natural immunity. They don't need the needle and they don't want it. Maybe they know something that bureaucrats and politicians don't.

The health care providers in Toronto have been given the same orders. Get the needle or be fired. A large number are going to walk away. Who then will keep the beds open during the fall resurgence? And the resurgence will come, needled or not. Look at what is happening in Israel. Already they are on their 3rd needle.

But in the middle of all this darkness and inexplicable incompetence, the Rubaiyat points out hope,

'Awake, for morning in the bowl of night
has flung the stone that puts the stars to flight,
and lo, the hunter of the east has caught
Scandinavia in a noose of light.'

When I was in Sweden I always thought of it as a dreary sodden place, like Ibsen's play Hedda Gabler, all depressed and suicidal. I do remember one wild week in Stockholm which I described in my book Have Knife

Will Travel. It was the first international conference for European artificial limbs and shoemakers, and it was great fun.

All Western medical knowledge and customs, garnered over the centuries, suddenly in 2020, on the advice of the despicable WHO and CDC, was suddenly thrown away. Sweden, essentially alone, remained as a beacon of sanity. All they did was follow the 2019 rules, and ignored WHO, as they were obviously pushing the orders of their CCP masters.

Sweden simply said, 'there is a bad respiratory virus on the loose, so be sensible.' Schools largely remained open, there were no crazy lockdowns or mandates, masks, or needles. Those merchants of fear porn, the computer modelers, claimed Sweden would die. They were as accurate as their global warming buddies. Karl Popper said, 'a single negative finding destroys a beautiful theory.' Sweden has done that. They have utterly disproved lockdowns, masks, and mandates.

What is hard to understand is the furious determination of the Anglo politicians and bureaucrats not to accept the reality that Sweden was right, and they were wrong.

The vaunted health care systems of the West, especially the US and Canada have failed miserably compared to El Salvador, Uttar Pradesh, a state in India, and other countries. They gave out for free, little packages of medicines which cost less than $10 and which cured the vast majority.

One looks on with horror at the totalitarian nightmare taking place in Australia and the runaway inflation in Canada. Venezuela South and North I guess.

But it doesn't have to be like this. Norway and Denmark are now following Sweden and removed all mandates. 'Just another bad flu', they say. So maybe there is hope, as the Rubaiyat says,

'Dreaming when dawn's left hand was in the sky.'

Q,1. Right on the money. This is crazy. We are sending our granddaughter to a private school so she can go in person with no mask. Her private school has no cases of the virus. That tells you everything you need to know.

Q,2, This is a nightmare story. There is no possible medical justification for this. So why are those in authority doing it? Following orders was not an adequate excuse at the Nuremberg Trials.

Q,3. FB is constantly taking me down when I try to provide information from my nursing contacts in Europe and North America, and any information from the nurses who are being fired. We have to stand together regardless of our vaccine status. If the nurses are let go, who will look after the patients?

Q,4. Even knowing the vaccination doesn't stop infection or transmission most people still want the unjabbed to be jabbed. It is almost as if their brains were turned off by that second needle in the arm. I am tired of this. Maybe it is time to go to Sweden.

A,1. What can one say? These are all highly intelligent women and their points are absolutely valid.

Q,4. A video has shown a molecular biologist who calls part of the mRNA needle a prion.

A,4. I listened and she did. She pointed out that there is no long term data whatsoever and called the whole sorry affair a Plandemic. When my coauthor Edna Quammie and I were looking for an easily controlled bioweapon, we elected to use prions. We knew that prion research was being conducted in that bioweapons lab in Wuhan. So we called our new book, 'Prions From Wuhan.'

October 6 at 6:35 PM

'Canada will be the country with the strictest needle mandate.' Thus spake Justine, the dear leader of Canada. A negative test will no longer suffice. If you want to do anything, a needle passport is required. 'All for your safety.'

Are he and his advisers really that dumb? Why do they ignore the evidence of Israel, the almost universally needled country? There the hospitals are filling up with the double needled, just as Knut and Geert predicted. The needle passport in Israel is now only valid after the 3rd or 4th booster as the needle prevents neither infection nor transmission.

The level of propaganda in Canada would make the CCP proud. I saw on my computer this morning a message from the U of Toronto. They claim 99% of students and staff have had the needle. That's so obviously untrue, unless there are a huge number of black market needle passports. How long would it take for one of these tricky computer kids to create one? Just asking. The U of T obviously doesn't believe its own propaganda as they are threatening job loss for all the un-needled, even if they are working remotely.

On my computer also this morning the hospital is begging nurses to sign up as they are desperately short of staff. The car radio was saying that hospitals across Canada are so short of staff that they are going to bring in the military. If that's true, why are they firing nurses by the thousands?

These nurses either recovered from the virus or were naturally immune to it. There is absolutely no medical justification for forcing the needle on these people and they know it. One feels humbled at their courage as they walk away into an uncertain future. As the poet wrote,

'the song of courage, heart and will
and gladness in a fight.
Of those who face a hopeless hill
with sparking and delight.'

These are the proud heirs to the Magna Carta, signed by King John at Runnymede on the 15th of June 1215. It read, 'To none will we sell, to none will we deny or delay right or Justice.' That was the proud heritage of the Anglo world. It is heartbreaking to see it being trampled into the dirt.

And then to realize you don't have the courage yourself. The phone-call in the night from the Chief of Surgery, 'if you don't get the needle, don't show up at the hospital.' The temptation is to say 'up yours'. But then to walk away from your life's work, from what was meaningful for the last 50 years. So you dutifully line up for the needle, realizing you would have been one of the bystanders watching the people being loaded onto the cattle cars on the road to Auschwitz.

It is always one step at a time. First they came for the doctors, then the nurses and other hospital staff, and finally the little children. It's OK to needle us older people as we will die soon anyway. But to needle children who have their whole life ahead of them, 'with hope like a fiery column before them.' They have already had almost 2 years stripped from their lives by this needless, foolish lockdown, and now this.

The health care system in Canada seems to be collapsing under the weight of contradictions. One is tempted to follow Jaroslav Hacek's 'Good Soldier Svezk,' and carry out every ridiculous order to its ludicrous conclusion. But while that might be satisfying, how does it help the suffering populace? So I guess we just struggle on, putting one foot in front of the other, hoping the nightmare will end someday. Even the monstrous tyranny of the Soviet fell in 70 years, although the CCP is still going strong.

So maybe we will just have to continue to,
'chase the rainbow through the rain,
and hope the promise is not vain,
that morn shall tearless be.'

Q.1. This is the weirdest time I have ever lived through- - - well, not through yet! I have never seen such a push for a new medical procedure, to be given to everyone regardless of need- - - just so weird. Wondering how long it will be before I starve to death once they no longer let me work.

Q.2. Sorry you were forced to take the jab. It takes a strong person to submit to something they are completely against, so my hat off to you sir, for taking the jab to continue to help people. For the last couple of years I have been thinking. Thank God I am closer to the end than the beginning. With that said. I have seen videos of nurses in tears saying they are taking the jab so they can continue to feed their children. I have also seen videos of nurses in tears saying they just can't do it and have no idea what the future will hold. I am dumbfounded that the medical community is allowing this.

A.1, What more is there to say? None of this makes any sense unless there is indeed an agenda. If there is, it surely cannot be good for society as a whole. But don't depend on doctors to speak up. They are easily cowed as they can lose their license, something they have dreamed of and worked towards for years, at the stroke of a bureaucrat's pen.

October 11 at 6:01 PM

Will the dreaded algorithm allow any discussion of mandates? If it does, when is a mandate not a mandate? I was listening to a bunch of lawyers this morning. In the US, some state AGs claim the mandates are not law. But in 2 cases recently judges decided that universities had the legal authority to mandate the needle, even in people who had recovered from the virus and had demonstrable antibodies. Clearly this travesty is Faucian logic at its finest and nothing to do with reality.

In Ontario Canada, the mandatory needle is apparently not a mandatory needle. It is mandatory for companies like a hospital to have a needle policy. But what exactly this policy must be is not clear. It is all 'Alice in Wonderland', or 'Blunderland.'

Our dear leader in Canada, Justine, is mandating that everyone have the needle, regardless of their immune status. Listening to a couple of employment lawyers arguing. They could not decide if staff who refuse the needle, with a perfectly good excuse, like a pregnant nurse who has recovered from the virus, would be entitled to severance pay or not. Another triumph of clear Public Health policy.

It is like a statement from the sainted Dr. If he states that green is purple in the morning, by afternoon he is claiming he is being misquoted.

There clearly is a shortage of healthcare providers in North America. This shortage will get infinitely worse as nurses who don't want or need the needle are fired. The governors of some states plan on bringing in the National Guard. But these people have full time jobs elsewhere. So it is bait and switch. Take a nurse from one hospital and transfer her to another. That hardly solves the problem, does it?

In Canada there is talk of bringing in the military to replace the fired nurses. Does that mean military nurses or soldiers acting as nurses? They did that in the nursing homes in Canada, and from their complaints, clearly the military had no idea what they were doing, and the difficulties of end of life care. Edna Quammie and I wrote about the difficulties and tragedies of this in our book 'Rainbow Through the Rain'.

Science, as a Western discipline, seems to be vanishing. It was already under siege with the advent of equity and inclusion invading the STEM fields. I mean, female glaciology?? The end was in sight with Climategate when the whole premise of Global Warming was shown to rest on phony data. The Roman and Medieval warm periods were concealed, and no one cared. The legacy media and politicians carried on blithely. The current utter failure of renewable energy, with the collapse of supply chains and the energy crisis in Europe and the UK may bring the failure home to people this winter when they can't afford to heat their houses.

If you can make the Medieval warm period disappear, then it is easy to conceal or deny natural immunity, and to label drugs, which have been in use for decades, as ineffective and toxic.

I am not against vaccinations. For 30+ years I traveled the world teaching and demonstrating modern joint replacement surgery. So I had every vaccine known to man. But these had a long track record and animal testing.

When my engineering colleague and I were developing porous metal, which is currently how most artificial hips and knees are held in place, I spent years doing animal testing before I put it in humans. And the metal was an almost completely inert cobalt / chrome alloy, not some bio-active stuff.

So of course health care providers are concerned about the needle, especially women who are pregnant or of child bearing age. There is no 5 year data. I mean maybe it's fine, but again- -.

I used to admire and defend big pharma but was becoming slowly disillusioned. In our novel 'Prions from Wuhan', Edna Quammie and I showed a little of the seamy side of that business. But this recent behavior has forced us to rethink their role, and they look increasingly like the villains.

Q,1. I don't understand this either. You are still just as likely to get the infection after the vax, so why push it? We're seeing many fully vaxed patients admitted into my hospital!

A,1. Exactly correct. Look at the data from Israel. It is not clear that the booster is doing much either. So what? Another booster. Will they fire all the nurses who don't get repeat boosters?

Q,2. This is crazy. My best friend is an online teacher and is being forced to get the needle. She is a single mom with no savings and doesn't have a choice. She has significant medical contraindications to the vax and is terrified right now.

A,2. Your right. It makes no sense. Why are they so desperate to needle everyone including poor innocent children with an experimental drug? Is it all about money?

Q,3. A judge has ruled that immunity after infection was not possible. This is ludicrous. It seems clear, even our judicial system can't remain impartial.

Q,4. The US National Guard has not yet been mandated to have the needle. So the unvaccinated National Guard will be replacing the unvaccinated nurses. Makes sense, eh?

A,3@4. None of this makes sense. It is hard to believe that even politicians would be so corrupt to do this purely for money. But what other explanation is there?

October 16 at 11:34 AM

Has the world gone mad? We have a worldwide manufactured disease tightly targeted at the ill elderly. Rumor has it that too many people in a certain large country were getting government pensions from a government no longer keen to pay for these unproductive people. I am sure that's a 'tin hat' theory, but so many 'tin hat' theories have so far proved correct. I still haven't seen lizard people on the streets, but maybe that's coming.

The Bat Lady of Wuhan had been taught in North Carolina how to juice up a poor harmless virus by inserting a furan cleavage site. In a CCP military lab, funded by the sainted Dr, she added SARS in 2016 or thereabouts. The real concern in 2019 was that she had added HIV, stolen from the level 4 lab in Winnipeg. That would have been doomsday for the human race as there would be no immunity, ever. It was then released or escaped during the Military games in Wuhan in the fall of 2019 and thus was spread over the world. It was given a major boost in the Chinese Lunar New Year when air travel inside China was banned and yet millions were encouraged to leave Wuhan to spread it to the rest of the world.

The virus, being seasonal, something we don't really completely understand, then triggered and the symptomatic cases went exponential. This was greatly aided in some places like New York by forcing sick people into the fertile ground of care homes.

Care homes are not hospitals. They are always under stress because the West in the last 50 years has refused to think seriously about the end of life. We will all go through the Gates of Death eventually. The question is not if, but how? Will we face it when we still have the cognitive ability to make decisions or will we let life slowly flicker out with the mind gone and the body still marginally functioning? These are serious issues. My coauthor and long-time scrub nurse, Edna Quammie and I looked at these problems in our book 'Rainbow through the Rain.'

The economic crisis in the West with coming runaway inflation will mean that in many cases the cost of Care Homes will be unaffordable. My mother looked after my parental grandmother in our home until she died. But who does that now? Who can afford to do that now when a double income is required to keep a roof over the family's head and food on the table?

Lockdown was actually a theory proposed by a US schoolgirl. But her model was a disease transmitted by touch, not an airborne virus. The CCP spread propaganda videos of trucks spraying clouds of chemicals in the streets, which would do nothing for a respiratory virus. All around us we see this obsessive cleaning with toxic chemicals which have no effect on an airborne virus. One wonders what damage all these toxins will have on kids.

Lockdown was pushed by these WHO officials who had no understanding of a Gompertz curve, which is certainly possible, as all they are is bureaucrats, or more likely were acting on the orders of their masters, the CCP. The computer modelers, who like their global warming buddies, are always prophesying doom, scared the Public Health Johnnies, who again are really bureaucrats, not docs, and politicians, who are lawyers and therefore know no science.

Lockdowns were originally ordered to save the health care systems from collapsing, which they never did, or were even close. By May of 2020 there was ample evidence that they were a disaster. So why did they continue? Another tin hat theory is that by keeping the mom and pop stores closed, the major donors to the politicians were making incredible profits.

The other question is why for the first time in the world's history were docs forbidden to use medicines which had been in use for decades? The excellent results from El Salvador and Uttar Pradesh were ignored. Who will shoulder the blame for these disastrous decisions?

And then we have this mandatory needle which neither stops infection or transmission, and yet without which all commerce is forbidden. Why is there this desperate push to needle kids who don't get sick with this virus and they don't transmit?

Am I missing something?

Q,1. I hear they found traces of the Nipah virus in that lab. Now that's a catastrophe waiting to happen.

A,1. I heard the same. They have apparently been working with that truly awful virus in the same leaky insecure lab. That one would make the Wuhan virus look like a walk in the park.

Q,2. I believe China achieved its goal of worldwide economic disruption, by the unplanned local escape after the controlled release at the military games. The fact of planned release was forecast by China ordering millions of PCR tests six months before the games.

A,2. The evidence seems increasingly to be pointing that way. Especially the new finding of the vastly increased orders for PCR test machines in the spring of 2019.

Q,3. I no longer know what to believe. I see the miracle vaxs apparently now need a booster every six months, for a disease which seems to affect the population more after the vax. Is this the population control they kept talking about in the great reset? I know it sounds crazy, but the worst of the conspiracy theories seem to be turning out to be true.

A.3. Who knows what to believe anymore? The theory about the boosters seems real enough. Our Dear Leader in Canada is boasting about the millions of vaxs he has just bought.

Q,4. I know it sounds crazy but I have heard that this virus is purposely designed and released for population control. There certainly were discussions about that prior to its release.

A,4. The Davos man, certainly made no secret that the virus was a good excuse to bring in the Great Reset, and Justine Trudeau in Canada loudly supported that.

October 20 at 5:20 PM

Kudos to the heroes! There are still some left. The Southwest Airlines pilots have beaten back the monstrous tide of tyranny sweeping over the world.

In the dark night of the soul, when you think all is lost, remember that the West retained its freedom, against all odds, at Marathon, Tours, Vienna, and led by Don Juan and his Italian admirals, at the battle of Lepanto. Tennyson's poem of that name which describes that battle is eerily like today,

'In that enormous silence
tiny and unafraid
comes up along a winding road
the noise of the crusade.'

But in those days,

'the Pope hath cast his arms abroad
in agony and loss.'

Sadly the current occupant is a pale shadow of Benedict and the Polish pope, who faced down the utter evil of communism.

But there are a few staunch men of God, like the pastor in Alberta who ordered the forces of the Antichrist from his church. For that action he is now facing 5 years in jail. Where is the groundswell of support for that brave man? Maybe a Canadian jail is not a concentration camp, but we need a few more Dietrich Bonhoeffers. He would say, 'first they came for the un-needled essential workers, then for the children, then for all those with only 2 needles; and where will it end?'

It was only a short time ago that the essential workers were being praised as heroes facing the fire of a new manufactured virus of unknown lethality. They did so unprotected as the CCP had bought up all the PPE, knowing that the plague was loose, possibly in May of 2019, and certainly by the October military games in Wuhan, when it was spread around the world. Being seasonal it didn't trigger until the winter of 2019, and then was really spread by the Lunar New Year diaspora from Wuhan. How curious it is that no country has had the cojones to ask China for compensation. Perhaps because the sainted Dr and his friends were funding it.

It is incredible that these bureaucrats, the Public Health Johnnies, and politicians, who were at no risk, sitting at home, never missing a paycheque, should now throw overboard those who faced the fire without complaint. Surely even the dullest and most corrupt, including the CDC, the FDA, and the rest, must know that those who survived are either naturally immune or have recovered from the virus and have far greater immunity than the needled.

I always loathed the FDA, as I wrote in my book describing how we developed modern artificial joints. But then I thought that they were just morons. But morons are occasionally correct and those in charge of the reaction to this virus have been consistently wrong. So now I think they are worse. I don't know what to believe. I know everything I was taught as a medical student about diet was completely wrong. I have since learned these food tables were made up by the food industry. So what else do I no longer trust or believe? Well, the cholesterol theory for one.

John Selden wrote in 1648, that the most abused sentence was. 'Salus populi suprema lex esto, or 'let public safety be the supreme law.' Nothing has changed in 400 years, and this sorry excuse is being used to justify endless, likely progressively more problematic, booster needles.

Q,1. This is a tragedy and mockery of health. Will those responsible ever be punished?

A,1. The Nuremberg trials were supposed to provide rules, but these are being ignored

October 23 at 12:34 PM

Reading O'Shaughnessy (1875) last night.

'Dreamer of dreams,

why should I strive to set the crooked straight?'

But then this morning rereading,

'for each age is a dream that is dying

and one that is coming to birth.'

Listening to Victor Hanson, the US historian, and one of the three originators of the Great Barrington Declaration. He cannot be named as he is persona non grata with the fierce algorithm and the mere mention of his name is the red rag to the collectivist bull.

He points out that the gift from Wuhan, if you look at the excess deaths year over year and country by country, is not much worse than a bad flu. It was, after all, tightly targeted at the ill unproductive elderly. If you compare country by country and in the US, state by state, the results are pretty much the same, and masking, lockdown, or anything else had not much effect. So if lockdown had no positive effect, then clearly it was a great mistake, a disaster. So who failed the world? There are numerous obvious groups.

The economists were silent. Many recent pundits of course are known for their collectivist ideology and so are merely shills. I found this out when I looked at my son's high school books. But Deaths of Despair is not a new term. Everyone knows that when there is an economic downturn deaths from alcoholism, suicide, and drug overdose skyrocket. Lockdown, by destroying the working class economy, was bound to increase these deaths. Since lockdown these have skyrocketed to about 100,000, mainly due to fentanyl, another gift from Wuhan. In the younger age groups more have died of despair than the virus. And no economist said anything to counter the Faucian deadly drumbeat of lockdown.

State education, especially in North America, played a significant role in the disaster. State teachers tend to retire early on gold plated pensions, so few are at risk on an age basis. By May of 2020, the data indicated that kids did not get severely ill and they did not transmit. So teachers were effectively at no risk, as they showed in Sweden, where junior schools never closed. And yet teachers unions, with their influenced politicians, fought to keep schools closed.

The children of the rich simply went to private schools, and the middle class kids had computers and tutors, but the poor kids had nothing, except this fig leaf of 'distance learning.' In Canada they kept the schools closed for 18 months. Will these neglected kids ever catch up? It has been suggested that this is very unlikely and that such children will lead poorer, shorter, sicker lives.

What was also ignored was child abuse. Most child abuse is identified at school. Distraught parents, with no job and no income, locked for months in an apartment with bored kids, what did they think was going to happen?

The General Medical journals ruined what was left of their reputation. The granddaddy of them all, Lancet, published a report that they must have known was fraudulent, as did many others. Most docs know that unlike subspecialty journals, General Medical journals are funded by big pharma. For the last few years they had been increasingly driven by those buzz words of the collective 'equity and inclusion', but I still thought they had some integrity. Now I simply look at the ads and toss the journal. They sound like CNN, the CBC or the BBC.

The medical bodies who control docs have equally shown their true colors. In medicine one size doesn't fit all. People are different so treatment must be tailored. And yet these bodies for no clear reason, stifled debate. In Canada they even went so far as to threaten doctors with loss of medical license. People ask, 'why didn't doctors speak up?' The threat of having all you have worked for all your life taken away by the stroke of a bureaucrat's pen is a pretty potent gag. There are not many Martin Luther's or Dietrich Bonhoeffer's in this world.

And the politicians, they have a responsibility to balance conflicting opinions. In many cases they abdicated, turning responsibility over to unidimensional, not too bright, Public Health Johnnies, operating on false data. In the fall of 2020, even the utterly corrupt WHO admitted lockdown was a disaster and yet it continued unabated in many countries.

The legacy media of course had been paid their 30 pieces of silver, so they did their masters bidding. But social media, even with all its ideologically driven algorithms, the corrupt fact checkers, and the like, is an unbelievable gift. To be able to listen to the finest minds in the world while walking down the street or working out is pure magic. So maybe O'Shaughnessy is right. 'A new age is coming.'

Q,1. Is there light at the end of this fabricated tunnel?

A,1. I would like to think so, wouldn't count on it.

Q,2. Southern California, of all places, is waking up. Our sports, adult leagues, are fully open outdoors and indoors- no masks. High fiving after the games. It's awesome! The doctors here though are still mostly asleep,...weird.

A,2. Maybe the world is waking up. The fired health care staff are suing. But I don't have great faith in our courts.

October 26 at 4:27 PM

The inequality of consequences! Everyone knows it exists, but who thinks about it? Driving back on the 401 superhighway in a rainstorm, listening to the car radio for traffic news. A new radio talk show host, was talking about 2 utterly incompetent ministers in the previous Canadian federal government remaining in the new cabinet. He pointed out that these guys are not fit to run a taco stand. But we all know that this is true of most politicians, especially sadly recently in our great neighbor to the south, and almost every federal minister of Health in every country in the world.

Jamil pointed out that this is also true for almost every bureaucrat, everywhere. It is the Peter Principle; they are promoted up to the level of their incompetence and can never be demoted or fired. In Yonge street in Toronto, one of the few arterial roads leaving downtown in a crowded, transit deprived city, the addition of bike lanes has reduced that street to 2 lanes, with no turn lanes. This, in a winter city where no one rides a bike for 6 months of the year! And yet, there are no consequences. We don't even know which dummy made that ludicrous decision.

So it is little wonder that this virus, which as DRASTIC has finally shown, was indeed funded by the sainted Dr, has been so mismanaged.

The Public Health Johnnies (PHJs), who are bureaucrats, most of whom never were practicing docs, believe in the Precautionary Principle, which basically is 'leap before you look'. They do one thing without considering the general implications of that action. Long before the Faucian gift from Wuhan, the PHJs in Toronto wished to slow traffic, which would certainly cut car impact deaths, but would destroy the economy and in effect, the city.

All the PHJs care about is the number of positive PCR tests. But we have known for over a year that this Drosten PCR test is fatally flawed.

Even the corrupt CDC now admits that it cannot distinguish from other corona viruses that cause the common cold, and even, dare I say, flu. The man who got the Nobel Prize for developing the concept, said it was never to be used in this manner. If you google his name you will find him describing the sainted Dr in terms of which many of us believe. I would definitely recommend listening. If you run the test at a multiplier of 20, then it may mean something, but in Canada we run at 42, which is about a trillion times and is utterly meaningless.

So why are we still doing it? There is clearly no medical reason. At about $140 per test someone is making a lot of money. I was always taught to assume stupidity before malevolence, but stupidity only takes you so far.

Similarly we have known for over a year that this is an airborne virus. So the videos from China of billowing clouds of disinfectant are for show only. This frantic deep cleaning with toxic chemicals serves no function other than making money for someone.

The videos of people dropping dead in the streets of Wuhan were very poor acting. People do not fall forwards with their knees straight and their hands out to cushion their fall.

I have spent a lot of time operating and teaching in China, and my wife is mainland Chinese. I don't know any Chinese people who would let themselves be welded into an apartment building. If you remember the Tiananmen Square massacre in 1989; the photos of the lone student standing in front of the column of tanks, you will understand why I don't believe any of these propaganda videos.

And where will this end? The next target is the kids. Not content with ruining their lives with lockdown, no school, no sports, loneliness, fear, masks, they are now coming after them with the needle. Who is 'they' and why are they doing it? It surely can't just be about money, can it?

As an essential worker I never lost a day from work, so lockdown didn't really affect me much. I was forced to take the needle last month or be banned from my hospital. But with the reduced age related immune response, at my age, the early effects are not much, if you live through the first month. They forced my 21 year old son to take the needle so he could attend classes at his university. This contravenes the code established at the Nuremberg Trials. So by international law, the bureaucrat who forced the needle on my son should face trial. But will that happen? Of course it won't. The radio host was right, the inequality of consequences will protect the bureaucracy.

Q,1. The Nuremberg Code is not international law.

A,1. I am not a lawyer, so I assume you are correct. But I did hear there was one case brought forward based on these principles.

Q,2. Some of these principles are to be found in various laws to do with human rights. I just wanted to make the point that the Nuremberg Code itself is not a law, although many think that it is.

A,2. So there you have it ladies and gentlemen. I guess it is not, but I wish it was.

Q.3. Sorry to hear you had to get the jab. But understandable to retain your license. My wife, who is a pharmacist also was forced to take the jab. She was sick for days after, as was another friend of mine. It certainly looks like this is all about the money.

A.2. I didn't want it, but given my age, I am not really at risk from a hyperimmune reaction. It is forcing the young people to take it which is a tragedy. As I understand it, older people need to be very careful for the first month or so as their natural immunity is temporarily severely damaged by the needle, or we hope the damage is temporary.

October 30 at 1:17 PM

'Do I really need to wear this dumb-ass mask?' asked the plumber, as he came into my medical office yesterday. Well no! Of course he doesn't. Let us consider some of the reasons why, most of which he already knows, being an industrial plumber.

Here is a guy who knows how to use a real mask, like a filter mask, when he is working in a building where asbestos is being removed. This is to prevent the tiny particles of one sort of asbestos (not all asbestos), from entering the lungs and possibly causing one type of cancer called mesothelioma. These particles are many times larger than the virus particles. No one who is working with asbestos, or a spray painter for that matter, is going to ever use a cloth or a surgeon's mask at work.

And somehow a surgeon's mask is going to keep out an airborne virus? Read the label on the side of the box the masks come in. On most it specifically states that they don't provide protection from a virus.

Think back to the start of this Plague. As I discussed in my book Journal of the Plague Year(2020), Canada was desperately short of masks, because for reasons never explained, the feds in Ottawa had shipped 7 tons of masks and other PPE to China in February of 2020. I found later that before the virus triggered in the spring, in countries like Italy and Australia the CCP had repurchased all the masks and other PPE and shipped them back to China. Much of this was later resold back to the same countries and hugely inflated prices. Smart businessmen eh? I guess somebody knew something. I think that is what we call 'insider trading.'

During this time the clerks in the grocery stores were dealing with hordes of people with no masks. And yet these grocery store clerks did not get sick. So why masks now? Who are the masks helping, other than those selling them?

Let us think a little more about masks. As a surgeon I have worn one all my life. The theoretical reason is to stop drooling into the wound. It is probably not necessary as there are studies that show the incidence of wound infection is not affected by masking. We change masks when they get wet, as a wet mask or a mask which has been wet and dried, allows all the facial and mouth bugs to be aerosolized and sprayed out. If you touch the mask with your hands then you contaminate it with whatever bugs are on your hands.

Masks must never be reused as the wet/ dry cycle simply encourages bug growth. If you really want to be horrified, then take one of your used masks to the lab and get them to grow the bugs they find on it. It is worse than washing your face in a public toilet bowl. You will have a hard time wearing a reused mask ever again.

And little kids are forced to wear a wet filthy mask all day! And someone somewhere is trying to pretend that this is good?

But we are not finished with masks. I find myself in the clinic walking past patients I have known and liked for years, hidden behind these obligatory masks. That's terrible for adult human interaction, feeding the epidemic of isolation and loneliness, and doubtless contributing to the huge increase in deaths of despair.

Children learn by interacting with other humans. If all they see are hidden faces, how can this not interfere with their development? In most countries in Europe, no kid under 12 is masked, as kids don't get sick with this virus and they don't transmit.

And the plumber and I have both, exceedingly unwillingly, been double vacd. Does the needle not work?

After I had fixed his wrist problem, the plumber was still seething with rage. His mother was in her late 80s in a care home. Every winter she got sick with a respiratory virus. As a dutiful son, he would spend day and night with her, expecting her to die. Last winter when she got sick, he was denied access. She died alone.

I saw in a recent video how the Amish handled this virus in their community. No one died alone. I have always liked these people as patients, and watching this video, my admiration grew.

Looking at an interview with an official high up in the last US administration. He has just released a book, and it turns out that the sainted Dr is even worse than I ever imagined.

Oh well! Look on the bright side. It is almost winter in Canada and still no lockdown.

Q,1. I live among the Amish here in PA, and fortunately for me, they never closed their businesses or schools, they don't do masks, and they don't run and get some stupid test every time they sneeze. I love my Amish neighbors.

A,1. They handled it with calm dignity. I bet in the final analysis they will be seen to have done far better than almost any other community.

Q,2. To my knowledge no one in their community has been hospitalized due to the virus. My husband drives them daily. They are such wonderful common sense people.

A,2. We don't have the Amish around here, but we have Mennonites who are very similar, admirable people.

Q,3. The Long March of communist subversion has been going on since the early 20th century. We are good at fighting conventional wars but are pathetically inept at psychological or cultural warfare.

A,3. That is my feeling too. As I outlined in the book I wrote with my long term scrub nurse, Edna Quammie, "The Big House,' we watched it happen in a major world class hospital, one tiny step at a time. Sadly we never found a hill worth dying on.

November 5 at 4:51 PM

Guess what! Met some really clever people last night. Needle passports all over but everyone ignoring mask mandates and social distancing. Inflation is clearly out of control as the restaurant costs were unbelievable.

I heard terrible stories from people I think know some things. Guess where and when the spike protein was patented; guess who sold it to whom; and guess who funded the development of the needle before the virus was released. I do hope that this was 'tin hat', but the details sounded awfully true. (Turns out they actually were.)

Leafing through a foot thick pile of notes I have been keeping since March of 2020. As information leaks out it looks worse and worse, frankly malevolent. Nothing is new I guess, William Shakespeare described it all 500 years ago, the sorrow and malevolence. In Macbeth,

'by the pricking of my thumbs
something evil this way comes.'

Or the tragedy of censorship with the suppression of information on medication which could have saved thousands of lives; and the utterly insane mandates locking up healthy people for months and ruining their businesses leading to uncounted deaths of despair.

The censorship, not only from the media, but also our overlords. In Canada we docs have been threatened with loss of medical license if we discuss the needle. We have instructions to follow the teachings of the CCP and WHO. Again Shakespeare in King Lear,

'the weight of this sad time we must obey,
speak not what we feel,
nor what we ought to say.
The eldest hath borne the most.

Those that are young
shall never see so much or live so long.'

As a child growing up in Scotland, I knew about the censorship behind the Iron Curtain. From popular fiction I knew all units of the Russian army had political officers, and that if an incorrect word was uttered, it was a bullet in the back of the head. I knew about the deliberate murder of the Russian army officers by Stalin, which left them ill prepared for the onslaught of the Wehrmacht. But I never imagined for a moment that the US military, the shield of the West, would decimate itself with woke politics and needle mandates. It is hard not to draw the inescapable conclusion of the enemy within or Lenin's 5th column.

Currently everything we do and everywhere we go is subject to government control and censorship. I no longer know what it is safe to write. In Scotland telling a joke or what you say inside your own house can result in criminal charges. Someone has said that it is the Anglo world which is under the greatest attack as that was the original home of the concept of individual freedom. Australia, New Zealand, and Scotland have fallen into the hands of the collective, and Canada is not far behind.

Rereading what I have written, it looks political. But as a follower of Thomas Jefferson's 'get off my lawn' teachings, I have always loathed politics. But most of us realized in the summer of 2020, when they introduced mandatory masking, that this inexplicable behavior no longer had anything to do with medicine.

Even the totally corrupt WHO, looking at the tragedy produced by the CCP encouraged worldwide lockdown, could no longer keep silent, and in the fall of 2020, denounced lockdown. And yet even in the face of this, countries like Australia and Canada continued. The blatant unfairness was obvious to all. The small businesses were closed but the multinationals stayed open. And the media and others claimed a scientific basis for this?

In a sense, I suppose it was. The scientific destruction of the middle class, the petite bourgeoisie, the backbone of a nation state. Was this the main purpose for the release of the virus, or simply a fortuitous offshoot?

Q,1. Attacks on small business and the middle class. So it seems. It makes me wonder if early viral events were intentional.

A,1. It sounds patently ridiculous, but what other conclusions can one draw?

November 10 at 1:33 PM

Double-think! Have you ever heard of it? It's a socialist concept. Indoctrination allows you to simultaneously accept two mutually contradictory beliefs as correct, often in contravention to one's own memory or sense of reality.

This morning at the hospital I opened my computer and was met with double-think announcements. From now on all people coming into my very large teaching hospital must show the needle passport. This includes my own associated little hospital where only hip and knee replacement is done, and so there are no sick people.

The next message was that there is to be an urgent meeting as there is such a shortage of orthopedic nurses that ongoing operations are in jeopardy.

Just for additional lunacy, I looked at the official medical journal from our masters, where they have decreed that docs in Canada must follow the guidelines of the CCP and WHO without question, on pain of loss of medical license. There is no mention in that journal of the collapse of the health care system. I have endless difficulties getting kids seen and the waiting lists for surgery are stretching out to infinity. These are not seen as serious issues. Instead the headlines are that docs must no longer tolerate bigotry in any form. Oh well, I am sure they mean well.

But returning to the double-think, surely by now everyone, except the legacy media and the Public Health Johnnies, knows that the needle neither stops infection or transmission. So the needle passport tells you nothing. And surely by now everyone knows that the infection rates of the needled are going through the ceiling.

Nurses, who worked through the epidemic, often with no PPE, and no medication, as such treatments were never publicized in Canada. Even the use of simple measures such as additional Vit D and C, zinc, and other natural products. Some were actually banned such as the two drugs who still cannot be named on social media. So these nurses have either had the virus and recovered or are naturally immune.

They know this as they are, after all, nurses. And so do hospital cleaners, secretaries, and the rest. Many are young women anxious to start a family or are pregnant. And these people are being forced to take a needle which has no long term studies. One can understand a certain reluctance, as news of adverse effects is being suppressed or at least made very difficult to report, even in Israel. So naturally they think the worst.

I mean maybe it will all be just hunky-dory, and a decade from now we will be holding hands singing Kumbaya. But it did take several years before the H1N1 vaccination was pulled off the market. Even I, a doc, only found out about the risk of narcolepsy last year, and I took that vaccine, fortunately with no side effects.

I have just seen that the CDC wants to impose masking forever, for the whole world. The Gauleiter of that tarnished institution, claims masking is 80% effective. If she actually believes that then we can stop needling, as after 4 or 6 months the needle is far less than 80% effective. But even that authority person of questionable loyalty can't actually believe what she has said. So why does she say it?

The mandatory needle I understand, that's big money. But masks? Does someone with friends in high places have a contract to supply masks? Just asking.

Q,1. There is something instantly questionable about official agencies worldwide pressuring all of humanity to take a particular medicine using uncommon authoritarian measures to force compliance.

A,1. Exactly! But why did effectively the whole world, except Sweden, fall into line? There were another couple of country leaders who didn't want it, like the man running Tanzania. They mysteriously died.

November 14 at 6:08 PM

'Just leave me the Fu- - alone.' A fascinating black swan event. Listening to Dave interviewing JBP, the Canadian philosopher. Dave was asking about the needle. P, struggling with other medical problems, was ill with the virus last year but recovered. Because people kept bugging him, he got the needle in Canada in the hope that the authorities would leave him alone. But this has not happened and he still has to jump through hoops to get back into Canada. His angry outburst raises all sorts of issues.

Firstly having had and recovered from the virus there was absolutely no need for the needle. The sainted Dr and his motley crew at the CDC refuse to believe in acquired immunity, a fact as old and as indisputable as time itself. Numerous studies have confirmed that post infection immunity is far more robust and long lived then the needle.

So there was no need for him to get the needle, which from the current hospitalizations it is clear neither stops infection or transmission. I know that some claim that it reduces the severity of the illness. Given the spike in death rates after the needle rollout in country after country such claims are not reassuring.

The third point is that P is young enough that he is not really at risk from the virus, which has a very steep age gradient. The adverse effects reporting is so suspect, even in Israel, that no one trusts the figures. Bismarck, the Iron Chancellor, who reshaped so much of our world, with concepts such as retirement, old age pensions, and universal schooling, said that 'nothing should be believed until it has been officially denied.' Docs joke among themselves that the official virus death rate should be divided by 10, and the adverse effects multiplied by 10. These are very conservative estimates. We docs in Canada have been forbidden to talk about the needle.

Another point driving P mad is this testing and quarantine on return to Canada. He has had both the disease and the needle so what is the point? Clearly the sainted Dr and the Public Health Johnnies don't understand or refuse to understand quarantine and test and trace.

The concept of quarantine comes from Venice, La Serenissima, the most beautiful city in all the world, the trade centre during the Middle Ages. Ships coming in from plague areas, the Black Death, had to remain at one of the islands in the lagoon for quarenta, 40 days. Once a disease is widespread within a country, quarantine is of no value.

Similarly test and trace is possible with a lethal disease transmitted by contact such as smallpox or Ebola. It is not possible with a highly infectious low mortality and morbidity airborne disease. I know that PHJs are not the sharpest nails in the box, but how difficult is it to understand that. These are facts as immutable as gravity. The millions of dollars wasted on these futile procedures makes one want to weep.

P is not an MD. He got the needle in the hope that officialdom would leave him alone. As the bureaucratic behavior remains unchecked, he naturally feels duped, a fool for allowing himself to be conned into taking the needle.

There are hundreds of hours of P's lectures available on YouTube, and he has repeatedly been interviewed by thoroughly unpleasant ignorant journalists. His motto is 'better to remain calm and let the unreasonable show their unreasonableness.' So to watch him blow his top gives a little hope that people will stand up to this insane despotism.

Q,1. Love P. Disappointed he got the jab though. It will never be enough for the ghouls.

A,1. He had to, otherwise he could not leave Canada. It is hard to believe that insanity, but it is true.

November 16 at 1:49 PM

Quiet day at the clinic so I looked up a 'black swan' event as I did not know where it came from. It is actually from Juvenal, AD 200, a Roman writer. His actual words were another phrase I vaguely knew. 'Rara Avis, a rare bird upon the earth, like a black swan.'

I noticed another one of his quotations which is as important today as it was then, given all these insane mandates and the threats from authorities to needle children. He wrote, 'sed quis custodiet ipsos Custodes? 'But who is to guard the guards themselves?'

And since I have always liked the ancient world, I looked up Euripides, 400 BC. He was obviously describing something similar to our handling of the Faucian gift from Wuhan, 'those whom the Gods wish to destroy, first make mad.'

The current madness is indeed destroying the West. But is it being done on purpose or because we have elected classic examples of the Dunning- Kruger effect? Hard to believe that the Dear Leader of Canada, and Brandon further south are capable of following a plan.

Q,1. We are losing our trust in doctors.

A,1. No wonder. But doctors are vulnerable. It is easy to take away their medical license, so they are very susceptible to threats. In Canada the threat is actually in writing. Many docs in the US, Canada, and I hear Australia have lost jobs and licenses for speaking out about the obvious absurdities in the handling of this tightly targeted virus.

November 18 at 5:21 PM

The year has almost ended so I am starting to edit book two of The Plague Year. I am thinking of calling it 'Plague or Pseudo-plague.' I would welcome ideas and suggestions. I added many of your insightful comments to the last book and would like more of your thoughts for this one.

A great medical clinic today, as usual. Old friends and new patients, friendly and laughing in spite of their problems. Most humans really are admirable. Makes one think of the War Poets.

'The song of courage, heart and will
and gladness in a fight.
Of those who face a hopeless hill
with sparking and delight.'

I feel so lucky to have stumbled into a job I love. But looking back, it is hard to think of a job I didn't like. As a boy I liked the physical work on the farms or in forestry. The only thing I remember not liking was General surgery and Neurosurgery. Spending hours inside a skull is utterly boring. But even that was offset because I had new and exciting research every evening.

So feeling great, then on the way home, I turned on the car radio. I really should stop doing that. The news is Canada is going to needle little kids. Why, oh why? What have kids ever done that these people so dislike them?

Those who wear a mask alone in their car are irredeemable. They are what Carl Jung called 'animus possessed.' There is no point in speaking to them. Similarly Public Health Johnnies (PHJs) are so deep in the mire they will never get out. But the rest of the world! Why? We have known since May 2020, that unlike regular flu, kids don't get sick with this one and don't transmit. I have yet to hear of a single documented case of a student infecting a teacher with this virus.

OK, needle the elderly if you must. We have only a few years ahead of us. But kids have their whole life. Maybe nothing will happen to most kids. Who knows? But we do know the risk of myocarditis, especially in boys, and who knows what will happen to girls 5 or 10 years from now.

I listened on the radio to a PHJ boasting about the good job they had done managing the virus. Maybe, but the worldwide figures of infections and hospitalizations don't seem any better or worse this year than last or the preceding years. And Norway has just released data showing no difference between the needled and unneedled in hospitalizations and outcomes.

I haven't seen Canadian figures, as with Australia we are lockdown central. But so far there is no data which shows lockdown had any effect, other than encouraging mutation escape and producing collateral deaths from cancer, strokes, and despair.

Austria has just imprisoned one third of its population. Israel is now saying that those with 2 needles are just as bad as those with none. The hospital where I have worked for 40 years insisted I get the needle. How long before they will demand the third? Should I tell them to do something sexually anatomically impossible, or should I accept the third, and then the fourth? And then what?

One hopes that K and G are wrong, but so far their frightening predictions have been correct.

Q,1. It looks like we are being played like a fiddle. It is bad enough to be fooled by a real magician, but the thought of being fooled by a bureaucrat like the sainted Dr. That makes you really feel like a fool.

A,1. It certainly is looking that way. I do hope not. I hate the thought of being the organ grinder's monkey.

November 20 at 11:37 AM

An upside down world. Macbeth described it. 'Fair is foul and foul is fair.' We all now know the needle doesn't stop infection or transmission. The Norwegian data indicates, contrary to what we are being told, if you are sick enough to need hospital there is no outcome difference between those needled or not.

New data also shows if you are needled, but not sick enough to stay home, you are a significant shedder of virus particles. So the needle passport does serve some purpose. Avoid those with it, as they are potential spreaders.

It is still assumed that in the ill elderly the needle gives some protection after the significant reduction in immunity for the first couple of weeks. But it is transitory. Those who got the needle 6 months ago have largely lost whatever immunity they had. Israel now puts such people back into the un-needled category. So they are on their 3rd or 4th booster. The UK is following suit.

Canada will soon follow as the Dear Leader has bought millions of needles for years to come. The kids will now be needled, for no clear medical reason, initially voluntarily, but soon mandatory to go to school. One zoo somewhere has just needled its animals. So domestic cats and dogs can't be far behind.

Listening to clever people talk about why respiratory infections are worse in winter. We cluster together indoors, and lockdown has shown that the Wuhan virus spreads in families in prolonged close proximity indoors. Central heating dries out the air, which damages the respiratory passages. So get out the humidifier. One wit pointed out that so does that test thing stuck up your nose.

The main factor seems to be lack of vit D. Writing such an obvious fact is dangerous as it alerts the censor algorithm. The federal minister of health in Canada calls Vit D misinformation.

I am not anti-vax, as having done a great amount of traveling, I had almost every known vaccination, as have my kids. But the definition of a vaccination was changed to accommodate this one. Ask yourself a question. 'If you were at minimal risk of a serious illness, would you voluntarily accept a drug which does not stop infection or transmission, has significant side effects, and needs to be taken every 6 months forever?' Just asking.

I seem to be writing a lot. But recently a cascade of information seems to be washing over the dam of censorship.

Q,1. I am not an anti vaxxer, I even got the shingles vaccine when I was able! But I see no value in this so-called vaccine. It does not stop you from getting Covid, it doesn't even stop you from dying from Covid as far as I can tell, with all the reports coming in from Ontario and other countries! I never saw a use for the flu shot either. When I was younger, both my daughter and I tried the annual flu shot for 3 years in a row. And for all 3 years we both got sick after taking it. That was enough for me to say no, no more shots of this nature. I have relied on my immune system since and I very rarely get ill with a cold and I have never been hospitalized for the flu. I take vitamin D starting in November, until the sun shines again in April. Such a cheap and wonderful way to keep healthy. Why doesn't the government announce these beneficial ways to the people instead of shot after shot of crap that doesn't seem to stop anything? I continue to be baffled by these mandates and what's worse, the people just blindly following along!

A,1. I agree. I took the flu shot every year because the hospital I work for mandated it. But that was a vaccine. It didn't work most of the time but did no likely long term damage. The populations of the West are starting to rebel, but as neither the legacy media nor the politicians are taking any notice, it may be 'too little too late.'

November 22 at 4:06 PM

'Curious and curiouser,' as Alice said in Wonderland.

Have you ever heard of Agenda 21? No? Me neither? As you all know in the spring of 2020 virtually the whole world turned insane.

We knew that kids didn't get sick with the Wuhan virus and didn't transmit. We knew that the Hygiene Hypothesis is real. Kids have good natural immunity and need to be exposed to multiple viruses to build further immunity. Lockdown, by preventing exposure, seems to have contributed to the rise of serious Respiratory Syncytial virus infections in kids. We knew that kids have to be socialized early in life by contact with other kids, otherwise a certain percentage will end up anti-social, with real problems in later life.

And yet we ignored all of this and kept schools closed, except in Sweden, where junior schools remained open. And then in the summer of 2020, universal masking was mandated, based on no science whatsoever. In Europe at least little kids were spared. But in Canada, where our dear leader is an ardent supporter of the Great Reset, kids as young as 2 were masked. Why? How could anyone possibly justify this? And schools in Canada were kept closed for 18 months.

I was looking around the net for some explanation of this collective madness, when I came across 'an old man in a chair.' I have heard him before and he always sounded emotional and a bit crazy. But a great deal of what he said has come true. This time he said that this is Agenda 21 in action. I had never heard of it, so I looked it up. I wish I had not.

The original document was drafted in 1979 by the Canadian largely responsible for the global warming hysteria, and Gro, the life-long card carrying socialist. It was adopted by the UN at the Rio summit in 1992. I always thought that other than Canada, no one ever took the UN seriously. But I found that most Western countries have accepted many of those recommendations. The energy crisis which the people of Europe will experience this winter is a result of this push for renewable energy.

When I first heard the Great Reset Davos man, I thought it was a joke with a James Bond villain. 'You will own nothing and you will be happy.' But guess what? That's Agenda 21.

Do you know that less educated people consume less, which is good for the sustainability of the planet? Me neither! But schools have been closed for no reason I can fathom.

This sounds crazy. But google Agenda 21. It is in writing. It must be a nightmare and I will wake up soon.

Q,1. I was told several years ago about Agenda 21.... I thought the coworker was crazy until I looked into it.....and it's believers are very patient and also persistent... it's complete lunacy.

Q,2. My girlfriend told me about Agenda 21 back in 2020. Everything has been in line with it! But you know we and she are just conspiracy theorists!

Q,3. It is sad that society seems unable to look beyond the screaming headlines and see truths and facts. Some have always been willing to destroy others for the sake of avarice and control. So here we are.

A,1. I really didn't want to believe it. I still don't want to believe it. It is hard to imagine someone as dim as our Dear Leader of Canada being part of a huge conspiracy. But what is happening is so inexplicable.

November 26 at 4:45 PM

'They are not long the days of wine and roses.
Out of a misty dream our path emerges for a while
then closes within a dream.' Dowson 1895.

It is sorrowful to watch civilization, or at least the Western part of it, walk over the edge of the abyss into nothingness. Maybe those intent on the demise of a certain percentage of the world's population will inadvertently take the rest of the world with them. This might be the answer to the Fermi paradox.

Enrico Fermi, looking up at the night sky and the billions of planets, asked 'where is everybody?' This needle might be the answer. Frost wrote that 'the world might end in fire or ice.' Yeah, or maybe as a result of a fairly innocuous manufactured virus.

Everything every real scientist, as opposed to these WHO, NIH, and CDC bureaucrats, warned about looks like it is coming true. Dr S warned about the cardiovascular effects of the needle. He was ignored, but a new paper seems to confirm his fears.

G and K warned about using a needle which neither prevents infection or transmission in the middle of an epidemic. They were afraid of immunological escape with humanization of the virus, and concomitant reduction of natural immunity. That ultimately the virus would be able to bypass any immunity left.

The Great Barrington group warned of the devastation of universal lockdown, and it has played out exactly as they said it would.

And yet amid all this bureaucratic induced chaos, there is no retreat. Instead the jackboots can be heard in the streets. The thunderous knock on the door at night. The forcible removal to the concentration, sorry, quarantine camps in Australia and New Zealand. My very elderly patients from Eastern Europe recognize the signs.

Listening to the politicians, it is frightening that in less than 2 years the wonder and glory of the Enlightenment has collapsed. Listen to them!! 'Our patience is exhausted!' 'None is safe until we are all safe, so we must needle children.' 'It is for your own good.' 'You unclean people, 2 needles are not enough. You must have more.' All for a needle which everyone knows does not stop infection or transmission.

Will sanity ever return? It did in East Germany in spite of the fact that one person in three was a government snitch. But now with facial recognition track and trace, will it ever be possible? Are the needle passports simply another nail in the coffin of freedom?

Q,1. The latest horror is that the sainted Dr is making arrogant pronouncements about inoculating babies. Having failed at everything, why is he still in charge of anything?

Q,2. Difficult to believe. Josef Mengele springs to mind.

A,1. What is even worse is that I just listened to G. He is deeply concerned that this will produce autoimmune disease in kids.

November 30 at 3:59 PM

Omicron! Ohmigod! When I first heard the name I thought that someone was joking. It is actually the 16th letter of the Greek alphabet. I should have remembered because I studied Ancient Greek in high school. But the 13th and 14th are missing from this table of named variants of the Wuhan virus.

It should have been called Nu as that is the 13th. And of course a Nu variant is necessary because most people are losing their fear of the virus and are now skeptical of leaders like the CDC and the sainted Dr. Other than those who wear a mask alone in their car, most people now realize that if they are under 70 and healthy they have a minimal risk of dying.

Sadly in most Anglo countries relatively effective, safe, cheap treatments are still banned so that the needle can be used under Emergency Use Authorization. Now that one needle has been cleared by the FDA, in-spite of the clinical trial not completed, hopefully there soon will be no reason to ban these drugs.

Other than the legacy media, big tech, the CDC and the sainted Dr, most people now know that the needle doesn't stop infection or transmission or, if the Norwegian data is to be believed, the serious effects of the virus. Most know of the side effects in young men and the long term concerns in young women. So we need a Nu variant to scare people into more needles before they exceed their best by date. But Nu was perhaps a little too obvious.

The next name should have been Xi, the 14th letter. That would have been entirely appropriate as the original virus came from Xi's city of Wuhan. Although it was funded through his buddies by the sainted Dr after such research was banned in the US. I believe such funding continues until 2023, unless Congress has banned it.

If the treating docs in South Africa are to be believed Omicron is an upper respiratory infection, like a bad cold. But according to the Public Health Johnnies the sky is falling and lockdown is back, and everyone, including maybe babies, needs the needle, again and again. I personally don't plan on losing any sleep over this variant unless the Dear Leader of Canada plans to follow Austria and make the needle compulsory.

But winter is coming in the North, so check with your naturopath. The fears that the non-sterilizing needle would lead to humanization of the virus with ultimate immune escape so far has not occurred. If it does then humanity will go the way of the dinosaurs. So keep your fingers crossed.

Q,1. Omicron spelled differently is 'moronic,' It describes the people already lining up for their shot. I haven't nor will I ever get the first one.

Q,2. The new Omicron arrived in Australia, so it was brought in by someone who is vaxxed, as the unvaxxed are not allowed in.

Q,3. Nothing says trust the science like 'you can't sue us if anything goes wrong.'

A,1. There may be an argument for needling the vulnerable, but the proof simply isn't there. There is no evidence whatsoever for needling the healthy under age 60 or 70.

December 5 at 6:43 PM

'Yea though I walk through the valley of the shadow, I will fear no evil.' I wish! Evil is a shape changer and comes in many forms. Currently it is disguised by the dreaded ever changing algorithm and by individuals of dubious loyalty who call themselves checkers of fact.

Currently in this era where people are afraid to speak aloud, I am not sure if it is safe even to whisper. But some brave scientists have put their careers in jeopardy by publishing their research and equally unbelievably, some medical journals have put their funding and very existence on the line by publishing. The whisper is that the needle has no effect on virus mortality. The whisper is also that in many countries there is no year on year excess mortality.

If so, where is the epidemic? Was it a mirage, a dream, or a man-made nightmare? Are we slowly awakening?

Sadly the merchants of menace and misinformation continue to trumpet their message from the rooftops. They continue to pump fear into those whose only source of news is the utterly corrupt legacy media and those fatally compromised bodies like the CDC, FDA, NIH, WHO and the Public Health Johnnies of most countries.

Many people are now beginning to understand that they have been fooled and are somewhat irate. Thomas Jefferson 1820, wrote that 'a little rebellion now and then is a good thing.' We are now seeing demonstrations all over Europe and the Anglosphere as a result of these disastrous mandates and lockdowns.

As expected, nothing of this is being reported by the legacy media. Again, as Jefferson wrote, 'advertisements are the only truths to be found in newspapers.' Maybe the groundswell of resistance to the needle will arrest the development of the needle induced humanized virus.

So maybe, in the midst of this immense unnecessary tragedy, it will be as Francis Thomson wrote,

'Halts by me that footfall.
Is my gloom after all
shade of his hand outstretched caressingly.'

Q,1. After almost two years of lies, when will the truth be told?

A,1. It has been told almost from the beginning, but it was smothered and those who told it were cancelled.

Q,2. The Premier of an east coast province has given permission for grocery stores to deny access to the unvaccinated.

A,2. Well, we knew it was coming. Some people from Germany have been warning that it feels like the 30s. Deja vu all over again.

December 11 at 12:07 PM

'Rejoice we conquer!' Or so I hope. These were the words of Pheidippides in 490 BC, when he ran from the battle of Marathon to Athens to tell of victory, that the West was saved. The Greeks had beaten back the Persian empire.

Listening to a statistician last night. Having published more than 200 scientific research papers, I knew that there were lies, damned lies, and statistics, but this was eye opening. He was reanalyzing UK government data on the virus. With a few minor adjustments he could show green is blue or blue is green.

He finally demonstrated that the needle had no effect on overall mortality, or essentially none. There was a fascinating sudden rise in mortality in the few weeks after the rollout of the first needle. I knew this was true for most countries. He made this disappear somehow, so clearly this man is not anti-needle.

His overall conclusions were fascinating. Firstly, the original needle trials, on which everything was based, showed nothing. Secondly, statistically speaking, there was no epidemic. It was nothing worse than a bad flu year. Thirdly, there is no evidence the needle is effective.

I checked again this morning and his lecture is still there on YouTube. So either the fact checkers don't understand what he was saying, which is certainly a possibility as their grasp of science is minimal, as they have just admitted in a recent US court case. Or they have accepted that his figures are accurate. If so, the party is over and we can all go home.

The other great news is that there has been an outbreak of the Omicron virus in Norway, and no one is severely ill. It is like the common cold as the original South African docs told us. So hopefully we have dodged the bullet of immune escape which terrified G and others. This variant seems more infectious and less deadly. If so, we need Omicron parties to spread it as widely and as rapidly as possible, so everyone can become fairly immune, just like the common cold.

Sadly the mendacious merchants of menace are never likely to accept that. Think of the money and power they would lose. Look at Israel. 2 needles no longer keep you out of needle jail, or is it 3 or 4? Austria and Germany are following suit. Australia and New Zealand have built concentration, sorry, quarantine camps. So watch for the next episode of fear porn coming your way soon.

Just a thought! Was that why they fired all the nurses and health care workers? Was it to produce a hospital crisis this winter? Do you have another explanation?

Q,1. Remember only a year ago when people were banging pots and pans to show our sincere appreciation for the dedicated docs and nurses.

A,1. Now they are being fired. Gratitude, eh?

Q,2. Two years after the virus release we should have enough stats and information to have really good information about it. Especially stats on the effectiveness of the vaccines, and other treatments. The fear porn produced by this new variant has raised the awareness of the incompetence of the idiots in charge.

A,2. Exactly. We are spending billions on that worthless CDC, and they have studiously avoided doing any worthwhile research on anything to do with the virus or the needle.

Q,3. Necessity is the plea for every infringement of human freedom. It is the argument of tyrants; it is the creed of slaves.'- - William Pitt.

A,3. And that is now the constant drumbeat across the West.

December 15 at 3:53 PM

'Fair is Foul, and Foul is Fair,' said the witches in Shakespeare's Macbeth. 'What is truth,' said Pontius Pilate. Today we face these questions, real, not rhetorical.

Was it always so? Was everything we were told a lie? Maybe it was, but I like to think not. But maybe I am just naïve and delusional.

I now know that what I was taught in medical school was frequently wrong. But I thought that was because we didn't know, not that we were being deliberately lied to. There were always suspect fields like diet, where the food industry played a role in disseminating misinformation, in exactly the same way the CDC, WHO, the FDA, and the NIH do today. The only thing I now believe about diet is to increase the protein, decrease the carbs, and if it is manufactured, don't touch it.

My own field of orthopedics I thought was reasonably clean. After all, you either can or cannot walk. 40 years ago we used to do awful things to young women's knees. But that stopped when the arthroscope allowed us to look inside. I detailed that story in the book I wrote with my scrub nurse, Edna Quammie. If interested google 'The Big House'. There is still some snake oil, but mostly it does no harm and is not getting worse.

So what brought on this angst? A general medical journal I looked through had an article urging the needling of children. The authors seemed to be industry shills. How could a formerly reputable journal publish this? It is known that kids with no comorbidities are at virtually zero risk from the disease and at some unquantified but real risk from the needle.

This plague has been around for 2 years now, and people have enough experience to know what is real and what is media fear porn. The people who wear a mask alone in their car are irredeemable. They are what the great psychologist Carl Jung called 'Animus possessed', lost permanently in their own delusion. If there was a genuine fear of this virus, people would do anything to protect themselves. There would be no need to mandate anything. It is now abundantly clear that all these mandated lockdowns, maskings, distancing, hand washing and cleaning had no positive effect, and had severe collateral damage. Already the lockdown deaths far exceed the virus deaths, in terms of 'life years' and have only begun.

The longer this insanity lasts, the more the children are at risk, not only from the needle, but also as a result of isolation leading to the Hygiene Hypothesis. They have not been exposed to other viruses and so have no immunity to diseases which do kill kids like flu and Respiratory Syncytial virus.

Maybe Omicron, by infecting everyone with mild cold-like symptoms, will save the day and finally stop the madness.

Q,1. There are fifteen new books that are on the market so you can learn all about Omicron. Since this variant was only named by WHO on November the 26th, these books were supposedly researched, written, edited, published, and marketed between November 27th and December 2nd.

A,1. Really smart people eh? Prescient, like those working on the vaccine in 2019.

Q,2. Governments did not help when they prohibited the use of the two medicines known to help fight this disease.

A,2. Such an action was unspeakable and unforgivable. How many people did they condemn to death? Will the dead ever see justice?

December 21 at 6:21 PM

Did you hear the one about--? It sounds like the start of a bad joke, and I wish it was. The ruler of the CDC has claimed that 'science' has shown that masking is 80% effective. The legacy media, that font of knowledge, believes her. If that's what she said then we can stop the needle as within a few months the needle is only about 30% effective, so multiple boosters will be required forever.

What she was actually trying to say was that masking little kids is effective. Eventually, an honest newspaper reporter, a true Rara Avis, thought that this sounded suspiciously like BS, and investigated. Guess what? It turned out that this was absolute junk science. The math was wrong, the number of kids in the study was ignored. Some of the schools were virtual, with no kids actually present. It was pure propaganda at its finest. It really wasn't fit to be used in a toilet. And yet the CDC stood by it.

Sadly this has been the standard of the CDC since the Wuhan virus outbreak. I thought that there were laws about truth in advertising. But these obviously don't apply to government institutions. And these people assure you it is safe and want to needle your kids.

No one in their right mind would believe anything from WHO after the CCP backed director with an exceedingly murky background took over. Sadly since May of 2020 it has become equally obvious that bodies such as the NIH, the FDA, and the like are equally flawed.

This group, spearheaded by the sainted Dr, have refused to accept any responsibility for lockdown, the worst public health disaster in history. The deaths and misery ordained by these uncaring bureaucrats is not I suppose unparalleled. The bureaucrats after all organized the Holodomor, the gulags, The Great Leap Forward, known in China as The Great Hunger, when 40 million starved to death, and even kept the trains running to the death camps while the German army was collapsing around them.

And now we have Omicron, where to date almost no deaths have occurred. And yet we have lockdown again. But this time with mandatory needles, soon for kids, babies, and pregnant women.

This last 2 years has truly been, dies irae, dies illa, dies calamitatis et miseriae. The forces of incompetence or evil seem all around us. But it is almost Christmas, Christ reborn. So pray for us now in the hour of our darkness.

December 23 at 5:35 PM

The year is almost over. A time for reflection. Just what happened? Most of us are too shell-shocked to know. That's a medical term from WW1, and is now called PTSD, Post Traumatic Stress Disorder. All of us, except for the lockdown supporting class, are suffering from it to some degree.

In the medical clinic I see daily the physical manifestations of depression and anxiety of people who have lost everything. Their job, their life savings, everything they worked for. All gone because of the incomprehensible and nonsensical orders from uncaring, unthinking Public Health bureaucrats.

It has been clear since May of 2020 that lockdown served no purpose and was the worst public health disaster in history. And yet, here it comes again. All because of the Omicron variant which has possibly killed 8 people in the whole world.

For the first time in living memory outside of Communist states, churches were closed and the comfort of their faith denied to sufferers. With a few heroic exceptions church leaders allowed this to happen. The ill elderly were forced to die alone, denied the comfort of their family and their God.

'That song whose singers come
with old kind tales of pity
from the great Compassion's lips.
That makes the bells of Heaven to peal
round pillows frosty with the feel
of Death's cold finger tips.'

And the children, our future if there is any. Locked away in the prison of home; no school, no friends, no sports, none of the carefree joys of childhood. In Canada the schools were closed for 18 months, in spite of the fact that we knew in May of 2020, that kids did not get sick with or transmit the Wuhan virus.

The kids in my clinic have complaints I never saw before. No wonder, sitting all day at a computer as they are allowed nothing else. They are weak, obese, depressed, and afraid. They are being threatened with this unnecessary needle and are again being told by the Global Warmists the world will end in 7 years. Those hypocrites who are scaring the kids with threats of rising sea levels are buying mansions on the seashore.

For most of us, other than the 'animus possessed' of Carl Jung, who can be recognized as they wear a mask alone in their car, there is a growing realization that what we are being told is not correct, and yet the politicians and PHJs carry on with the same disastrous failed policies.

But the winter Solstice has passed and the days are getting longer. I guess while we live there is hope.

Q,1. The PHJs and bureaucrats have gotten us attuned to lockdown and other restrictions, so that is not likely to change soon. The Military Games in Wuhan in 2019 were possibly a test drive for a virus release. What new virus will the CCP gift us by infecting the Olympic athletes?

A,1. I never thought of that!

December 27 at 10 PM

'Look Back In Anger', was the title of a play written many decades ago. It wasn't very good, but the title accurately describes the chaos, lies, and mismanagement of the last 2 years.

Tennyson wrote about the new year,

Ring out wild bell, the year is dying in the night.

Ring out wild bells, and let him die.

Ring out the old, ring in the new.

Ring out the false, ring in the true.'

But sadly there is little sign of anything new or true in this desperate fight against the common cold, sorry, Omicron variant. To date, in spite of the world wide panic, only a handful have died, but with or of the virus?

This new iteration of the virus has produced spasms of delight among the politicians, legacy media, and PHJs. These Gauleiters seem to have a perverse joy in ruining the lives of their fellow humans. They seem bound and determined to re-implement all the old utterly failed policies of the last 2 years. Let us briefly consider these manifest failures.

Universal masking was always silly, as anyone who ever wore a mask at work knew. Plexiglass everywhere was just stupid.

There was no scientific basis for distancing. Obviously a large crowd jammed together indoors does not seem like a good idea, but in reality, nothing has happened.

Testing with the PCR, at 97% inaccuracy, was always pointless and should be stopped. Asymptomatic spread was very unusual.

Test and trace was pushed by those who clearly had no idea what they were doing, as it was never possible with a highly infectious low morbidity airborne virus. And even if it was, the fact that in most of the world no outpatient treatment was offered made the whole exercise pointless.

All this frenzy of cleaning with toxic chemicals for an airborne virus never made sense. Mom and pop stores were closed on no basis, as were restaurants, nightclubs, and gyms. Places where sick people don't go.

We are still not able to talk about the needle, although more and more docs and scientists are beginning to voice their deep concerns. The least needled countries have the least cases. Corrclation doesn't equal causation, but, but!

Anyway we pray for sanity and for freedom in an unfree world.

Have a good New Year!

December 29 At 5 PM

I thought I was done for the year, but this is too delicious not to report. Quebec, Canada, the sub country which is vying with Victoria, Australia, for the lockdown and mandate capital of the world, has run out of nurses and docs.

As Chaucer wrote in 1390, 'the greatest clerks (bureaucrats) be not the wisest men.' First the Quebec bureaucrats fired all the nurses, who for perfectly valid reasons, such as natural immunity or pregnancy, refused the needle. A couple of months ago, they realized they were short of nurses so they offered a $15,000 signing bonus for retired nurses to return to work or to switch to full time. That did not help, so today they announced that those testing positive from the virus can continue at work and do not need to quarantine. Oh the irony! Bureaucracy at its finest!

The other good news is that the current US federal government has finally realized that the US is a federation, and that all states are different, not only in geography, but also in population, etc. Decisions about a seasonal virus must therefore be made at the state level. A universal policy makes no sense.

Now if only the PHJs would listen to Sweden or Florida, sanity might return to the world. But there is no sign of this. William Cowper 1780, wrote that 'a fool must now and then be right by chance.' But there is no sign of that in the CDC and others. It is almost as if Francis Thompson was thinking of sanity and commonsense when he wrote the Hound Of Heaven.

'I fled him down the nights and down the days,
I fled him down the arches of the years.
I fled him down the labyrinthine ways of my own mind'- - - -

But I do hope when the next year comes that it will be as Francis Thompson wrote,

'halts by me that footfall, is my gloom after all
Shade of his hand outstretched caressingly.'

Envoi

And so the year ends as it began, with a quotation from Shakespeare's Julius Caesar, 'a year older, and no wiser, and the crowds along the Appian Way remain the same.'

We hoped at the start of 2021, as the US legacy media, various governors, big tech, and the rest of the passionate warmists and globalists had achieved their stated objective of unseating the US president, that sanity would return. We had at that time only a glimmer of an idea of how corrupt agencies like the CDC, NIH, and FDA had become.

Sadly every move by all these groups saw one nonsensical edict after another and liberty become more constrained. Freedom became something promised by the elite, perhaps some time in the future if we were good serfs and obeyed our masters. One mandate after another was imposed, based on no science whatsoever or even common sense. Public Health Bureaucrats, whose grasp of medicine, and even reality, appeared to be sadly lacking, became the face of science.

Censorship intensified. Repurposed drugs, whose safety had been established decades ago, were banned. Considering the success of these drugs in countries as separate as El Salvador and Uttar Pradesh, those who banned these drugs should forever feel like Lady Macbeth,

'Will all great Neptune's ocean wash this blood from my hands.'

Any discussion on alternative treatments was forbidden. Sensible recommendations regarding weight loss, sunshine to provide vitamin D and treat light affective disorder, and a return of children to school did not take place. Instead there was this constant drumbeat of vaccination even in people who had recovered from the virus and therefore by any sane definition were immune.

This absolute and unimaginable refusal to accept post-infection immunity will be forever seen as one of the greatest blots on Western medicine. No serious person accept and promulgate this obvious ridiculous position for a single moment.

The gradual encroachment of forced vaccination, with a drug which until recently would never have qualified as a vaccine, continues. And this is in spite of the now common knowledge that it neither prevents infection or transmission, and in those who require hospitalization, recent data from Norway suggests no effect in serious cases. The immediate complications may be few, but are real and have been very poorly documented, as attempts to report adverse effects of the vaccines are extremely time consuming and difficult. The long term effects of these interventions are totally unknown.

At best they will be relatively ineffective but do little long term harm. At worst, vaccination with a non-sterilizing agent in the middle of a highly infectious low morbidity virus epidemic will lead to humanization of the virus with complete natural immune escape. If that happens, then Fermi's Paradox is answered. Looking at the night sky and the billions of planets he asked, "where is everyone?' Maybe suicide is the fate of all nascent civilizations. I hope not.

So will next year bring sanity? Given our current political leaders and their advisers, probably not. The recent moves of the EU are frankly terrifying, suggesting more mandates and restrictions to come. The advent in the last few weeks of Omicron, a new variant, has reduced the Public Health Johnnies, legacy media, and politicians to spasms of fear and further lockdown. And this is in spite of the almost complete lack of any deaths directly attributable to it.

Further lockdown is liable to complete the destruction of what was left of the petite bourgeoisie. Given that it is now common knowledge that lockdown produces no positive effects and endless tragedies, it's continuation is so inexplicable that one is left wondering if this was the ultimate objective of the exercise. Perhaps the chaps wearing the tin foil hats were in fact correct. One sincerely hopes not.

It is becoming increasingly likely there will be another book coming out next year documenting the ongoing aching tragedy of this utterly mishandled, none too serious virus, tightly targeted at the ill elderly. Perhaps by then the true underlying motivation for this disaster will be obvious.

Acknowledgements

There are numerous quotations, not all entirely accurate, from sources as disparate as Cicero, Juvenal, and the Bible. The poetry is from Rudyard Kipling, Lord Tennyson, Kit Marlowe, William Shakespeare, John Donne, Francis Thomson, Sir Henry Newbolt, W.B. Yeats, the Browning's, Elizabeth, and Robert, and given the similarities of the current situation to the disaster of WWI, the war poets, Wilfred Owen, Rupert Brooke, Evelyn Underhill, the Hodgson's, Ralph and W.N., Siegfried Sassoon, A.E. Houseman and others.

CPSIA information can be obtained
at www.ICGtesting.com
Printed in the USA
BVHW031607140222
628721BV00002B/5

9 781669 810636